FAT WOMAN ON THE
MOUNTAIN

How I Lost Half of Myself
And Found Happiness

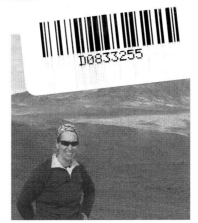

A Memoir

KARA RICHARDSON WHITELY

www.fatwomanonthemountain.com

Fat Woman on the Mountain:
How I Lost Half Myself and Found Happiness
© 2010 by Kara Richardson Whitely.

For information address:
Fat Woman on the Mountain
PO Box 774
Summit, NJ 07902-0774.

Fat Woman on the Mountain Website:
www.fatwomanonthemountain.com

10-digit ISBN: 1-451592-32-9
13-digit ISBN: 978-1451592-32-0

Cover and interior design by Leeza Hernandez
www.leezaworks.com

DISCLAIMER:
Kara Richardson Whitely shares her story about what has worked for her.
She is not a physical trainer. Before starting a weight-loss plan or physical
activity, check with your physician to make sure your plan is right for you.

Some names and identifying details have been changed to protect privacy.

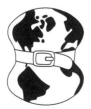

For Chris
My husband and hiking partner

CONTENTS

INTRODUCTION

My chest rose, hoping for oxygen, but sunk like a disappointed balloon as I neared the summit of Kilimanjaro.

Every day of my year-long training, I had imagined being there, posing in front of the crooked summit sign bidding "Congratulations" and "Welcome" on the wind-whipped snow.

My eyes welled, spilling tears that quickly went from warm, salty syrup to cool streaks down my cheek. I had hiked Africa's highest peak-all 19,343 feet of it. Even though I could barely inhale the thin, dry air that comes at such altitude, I smiled with chapped lips knowing I survived.

When I was 120 pounds heavier, I would have settled for standing in the cold comfort of an open refrigerator, searching for something to saturate what I was feeling at that moment: happy, sad, fearful, lonely, anything. I'd even clink through the condiment shelf, seeing if there were any maraschino cherries left. I'd eat anything to feel nothing.

This is the story of my journey up mountains and down the scale.

I was fed up with paying for weight-loss programs each week but not following them, hearing about the wonders of stomach-stapling surgery, being bombarded by metabolism-enhancing pill ads, and buying the "diet du jour" books that I'd start and quit almost as fast as I cracked them open. I hated the idea that I was a failure if I didn't go from fat to skinny in one diet alone–so I made mountain hiking my weight loss plan. I went to the woods because I had stopped living. I had become an all-black-wearing, thigh-chafing fat girl.

I was lost within my own body but found myself on the trails. This new path led me to the top of some of Vermont's highest peaks, including Camel's Hump (twice) and Mount Mansfield. I've also been to the bottom of the Grand Canyon and (thankfully) back up again.

I felt stronger with each step, so the following New Year's Day, I decided to join Global Alliance for Africa's fund-raising trek up Kilimanjaro, the highest freestanding mountain in the world. It's also the highest mountain one can climb without ropes, supplemental oxygen, and ice axes (that is, assuming all goes well).

It was on this six-day journey (five days up, one day down) when I learned that mountain hiking, particularly on Kilimanjaro, and getting healthy have a lot in common. They require tenacity, determination, and faith.

You keep trudging along minute after minute, day after day, and sometimes after miles and miles of walking in the dense forest you have no concept of how far you have come. You think about turning back but you don't want to go back on that trail again. Then at last, after a long, hard journey, you reach your goal.

The path to wellness is full of peaks and valleys. It is a journey that lasts a lifetime.

1. INTO THE WOODS

The yard where I grew up in Canada was a forest. The velvet evergreen branches stood tall on studded trunks above patches of trilliums, the white and pink star-like flowers I'd tromp through with my older brothers Bryan and Derek. We lived in a winterized cottage along South Lake, a Thousand Lakes community where most people had summer homes.

Our driveway was a mile long. In the winter, the snow would sometimes accumulate as high as my five-year-old shoulders; my father would rev up the snowmobile and take us up a hill to the school bus stop. It was a perfect remote setting for my father, who was a Vietnam veteran.

I would follow my brothers' nature adventures over rocks and rusty pine needles in the woods. We three towheaded blonds swam in the lake, with pikes sometime nibbling at our toes. We'd look for salamanders in streams. Bryan, my oldest brother, was especially good at capturing the slimy creatures, only for them to escape and dry up in our home. Giant dragonflies rested on Derek's shoulder.

I'd run breathless, laughing, trying to keep up with my beloved black and white mutt Felicity. Nobody else liked Felicity much. She ate my mother's tulips.

My mother, a registered nurse who embraced more holistic medicines such as healing touch and other energy therapy, loved the back-to-earth lifestyle. She baked her own bread and canned her vegetables. After all, she had a vegetable garden the size of a football field, where peas curled around the vines and plump tomatoes were hoisted by chicken wire. We hoped the strawberries would turn out just right because that meant we could prepare a big batch of jam that would last us through the winter season.

The only hot dogs and sweets we ate were at friends' houses, especially at Danny's. Danny's teeth were rotted and brown. We had lots of friends for birthday parties and play dates. Lianne, who was a true beauty, was my best friend. I especially loved going to her family's lakeside camp because they kept every kind of soda I knew of in the cellar. When we drove there together, cases rumbling in the backseat, I couldn't stop thinking about which soda I'd have first.

If a sweet tooth is hereditary, mine came from my father. Once, my mother and my brothers went on a trip to California. She left Dad and me with individually marked Tupperware containers of dinners (spaghetti with homemade sauce and such) for the week ahead. One night, we skipped the ready-made meal so he could take me into town for hamburgers and strawberry ice cream. The ice cream was a perfect, girly pink with cold frozen strawberries that crunched as I bit down.

My father, ever-the-gadget guy, soon bought Mom a home-made-ice-cream maker. We took turns cranking it by hand as the ice cream cured in a frosted vault, surrounded by rock salt. It made me so happy.

Shortly after I turned nine, we moved to upstate New York so my father could study for his PhD. Our new home in

Winthrop came with more than seventy acres and should have been a naturalist's playground. But my home felt different.

Something wasn't right with my parents. Mom would cry into the phone. Dad would yell. I often found myself in the pantry.

One time, I snuck in the stale, dark closet before their confrontation spilled into the kitchen. I don't remember what they were fighting about. It was in the months before their divorce. It certainly wasn't about anything good.

I must have sounded like a mouse, fingers scratching, pulling, and peeling at a can in the dark. That is, if they could have heard me in between their mutual accusations.

I had to get in that can. I had seen it earlier when my mother unloaded groceries from tall paper bags. It was a small cylinder. On the outside there were pictures of bakery-perfect pastries. I wanted all of them.

I pulled off the plastic lid and tried to lift the metal tab. I gave it a solid yank, creating a ripping sound. My mother, who must have heard it, cracked open the door, shedding light on my sneaking.

I looked down and said, "Nuts!" In the light, I realized that I had opened a can of walnuts. The pictures of all those photographed confections were what one could make with walnuts, not what one could immediately pop in her mouth upon opening the can.

My parents seemed pissed. I was mad that I didn't get brownies.

Things didn't get much better in that house.

About nine months after moving there we took my things, my brothers' things, and my mother's things and packed them tightly in her station wagon. I held my father in a hug on the front porch, begging my mom to let me stay with him. My mother moved us to Vermont, where she had taken a job as an evening nurse and would finish her nursing degree.

In South Burlington, a wealthy suburb where doctors from the nearby medical center made their large homes, we rented a condominium at the bottom of a hill.

Cooking "au natural" wasn't so easy for Mom as a single mother. She came home from the market with instant macaroni and cheese, sugar cereal (perhaps to abate my tantrums in the grocery store), and all sorts of items I had envied in my friends' cupboards.

Within the first hours at my new school, it was time for recess. To my fourth-grade delight, I saw monkey bars.

I remembered this playground contraption that my friends and I would hang from and climb across with ease when I lived in Canada. I hadn't been on one during my entire time in Winthrop. I headed to the monkey bars with visions of better days.

I climbed the metal ladder-like steps to reach for the first bar. As I grabbed the first paint-chipped rung, it seemed farther than the last monkey bars I'd been on. I pushed off, using my tiptoes, to swing the second hand to the first bar. Suddenly, I realized I had gained a lot of weight.

Teeth clenching, I held with all the strength I could. My hands were sweaty, as my arms felt that they would separate from my shoulders. Now instead of trying to swing to the next bar, I wanted to go back. I was frozen there. My cheeks puffed out as a mini-panic attack took hold. I wanted to scream for help, but didn't want to draw attention to the chubby kid paralyzed with fear on the playground. Besides, nobody knew who I was.

It was too late. In my indecision, my fingers were losing grip as my body felt heavier than ever before. I fell with a thud, knocking all of the wind out of my chest.

I landed just inches away from the concrete mold that held the monkey bars in place. My new classmates circled around me. Some giggled as I looked up dazed before being escorted to the nurse's office.

I told the staff I wanted to go home. I turned into a sobbing mess as soon as my mother came in the waiting room.

My first day at school ended early.

I ate and ate and became increasingly fat. The bigger I got, the smaller I felt.

I made friends with a classmate named Cam, who had a great ranch house, a big family with a mother, father, sisters, and brothers-and a huge freezer loaded with ice cream in the garage. Cam was adopted from Vietnam. So, in a way, she was different from everyone else, just like me. I wanted to be at her house every day—it felt full.

I wanted to dress "cool" like Cam and line my walls with all of the same pop star posters. Instead, the only place my mother could take me to shop was the plus-sized clothing corner at the department stores. My summer dresses never quite looked right. I bulged right out of lilac shorts, the elastic cutting at my waist.

Cam dropped me for the more popular crowd when we got to middle school.

I felt different. I was the only girl in my sixth grade gym class who topped one hundred pounds during the annual weigh-ins. The mark held on a manila card felt like a failing grade. I heard a classmate talking about my weight in another bay of lockers.

I had food. My cousin Tom, who would hang out at our

house, had booze. He also had a close clique of kids from broken homes. He was the soft-spoken tagalong of the group. Together, in their first few years of high school, they delved into drinking, sneaking beers from their fathers' stashes. I remember a few calls from the police.

Then there was our neighbor Darren. He was a dark-hearted fellow. For fun, he launched records like Chinese throwing stars across the room. The only person he aimed at was his mother, though he didn't have great aim. Tom often had to duck.

During a fort-building snow day in our neighborhood, my brother Derek made the mistake of throwing a snowball at Darren. Darren pummeled Derek and broke his nose.

That was nothing compared to the way Darren treated his sister. Even though Darren was older than Tom, his sister and I were the same age. I felt sorry for her and I tried to intervene. Once.

We went to their house, a disheveled ranch, and Darren was again terrorizing his sister. She ran room to room. When she slammed the door to escape, he'd pound on it, practically pushing his fists through the thin wood barrier.

I screamed at him, begging him to stop. He threw me against the wall, and knocked the air out of me. I tried to avoid him after that.

Even though Tom's clique sometimes brought trouble, I was a little jealous of their camaraderie. In sixth grade, my joys were lasagna day or extra tater tots.

In the wide open cafeteria, I wanted to sit on the corner bench-out of the way of the popular kids. Nevertheless, I wanted so much to be one of them. I even tried smoking, hoping someone would catch a whiff of my coolness, but I couldn't make it through a cigarette without going into coughing fits. It was middle school torture-being tormented by the very people you hoped would befriend you. Once, an upper classman passed me a folded paper, ripped out of a notebook.

I opened it: "Will you go out with me?"

The note was signed "JP," a cute, popular bookish boy in the seventh grade. For a moment my cheeks blushed and my heart swooned. Then, in a crashing halt, I recognized the same handwriting as other taunting notes from Clarissa.

Clarissa, a seventh grader, and her adolescent cronies who dressed in designer clothing, fed off my intense loneliness. She would send faux love letters from three lunch tables away, making me think that boys liked me.

She'd get me every time, at least for the first few seconds. I wished someone who liked me would send notes to me. Then, I'd hear giggles and slaps on the cafeteria tables and I knew that it was just a cruel joke.

I had never been on a date before. I went to middle school dances alone. I would try to break into dance circles in the streamer-laced cafeteria, even if it was to have someone to stand next to and shout out the lyrics to Billy Idol's "Mony, Mony." I tapped boys, all the boys, for slow dances. They all said, "No."

When the lip-sync contest was announced, I immediately signed up. I was the only solo act but made it past the auditions and onto the stage for the show. Not bad, I thought, since the other teams had parents make props for them.

There were no props in my act. I wore a long-sleeve red shirt with silver sequins. My mother let me use her lipstick.

My mother only had stacks of vinyl records from artists such as Simon and Garfunkel. She ruled out Olivia Newton John's "Let's Get Physical" because she said it was too racy. I thought it was about exercising. So I went to my neighbor's house because they had a more modern collection of cassette tapes.

They offered me the Flashdance soundtrack. We decided Irene Cara's "What a Feeling!" was a winner. I hadn't actually seen Flashdance, so my solo act with mere sidesteps to the beat on stage may have been out of context.

On the night of the show, while some kids gathered together in the cafeteria to get ready, I waited with my mom. I was so nervous I told her to come an hour earlier than we needed to be there. I spent the time remembering lines I needed to mouth: "Take your passion/And make it happen."

My thoughts were interrupted by the familiar snickering of Clarissa and friends. They laughed about me standing there with my mother. I snapped-and rushed toward her, fists flailing, and knocked her to the ground.

I finally gave Clarissa a chance to feel humiliated. She lay on the floor getting blow after blow from a girl who would normally shrug off her abuse. She never bothered me again.

I never got into trouble for that fight, even though I know the vice principal was in the school that night. He knew how she tormented me, and perhaps agreed she had it coming. I went on to lip sync my heart out on stage but didn't win a prize.

While fighting back may have ceased the barrage of insults from Clarissa, I still was an outsider. I wanted so much to be cool and have my own friends. As my twelfth birthday loomed in June, I ran the idea of throwing a party of "after-school-special" proportions by my mother. She turned me down, saying we didn't have the money to fund such a fest. It was enough to keep up with the rent.

No worries, I thought. I'd just have a gathering in the woods off the side of our condominium development. It was a path that

I had wandered many times without running into anybody. Surely there would be no one there at night.

I set it for the weekend before my birthday, an early June event that people would remember through the summer.

I was on the fringe of Darren's sister Donna's clique, which centered on the tall Berta. Berta was bordering on being a big girl. Her older sister was very heavy. I didn't get the sense Berta liked me very much. So, when I told Berta that I wanted to invite everyone, especially the popular people, and she told me that she'd take care of it, I was surprised.

I unveiled my plan to Derek and his Icelandic exchange student friend, Harolder. They cautioned me about an unsanctioned event, but I went ahead with it. Soon everyone in school was telling me, with a half smirk, that they'd be there. Finally, I would have friends.

It began on a perfect summer evening. Berta and her older sister, whom I'd never met, arrived with alcohol. I wanted no part drinking so I skipped a sip. I just wanted people, so I waited for them. An hour passed.

"Did you give people directions?" I asked Berta.

"Yes."

"Did you say the right date?"

"Yes."

Again and again I asked Berta. I was expecting the entire school, and I had Berta. Finally Berta fessed up, laughing, that this was a big joke. She had told people to tell me they were coming to a party-but they wouldn't. There was no party.

There in the woods that day I was so mad, so embarrassed— but I hid it. If I acted infuriated, it would have been funnier to everyone she would tell. She and her sister decided they wanted to skinny dip in the pool at my condominium development.

Then, someone did show up. It was my mother.

Derek and Harolder had driven off on their BMX bikes and tattled. They were afraid that I would be over my head and taken advantage of when all of those people came to my party in the woods. They were right. I didn't know what I was getting into.

It was the eve of my twelfth birthday, and I was spanked and grounded. No matter, I didn't have any friends anyway. There would be no party.

I spent my birthday watching television. It was the closest thing I had to company most days, anyway.

As I lay on my stomach, the nubs of carpet stuck into my legs. My side was cushioned by the living room couch. Tom came over to our house with Darren. They went upstairs together, but a little while later, Darren came down alone.

He sat above me on the couch. Suddenly I felt a foot, pressing between the back of my legs. I thought he had made a mistake. He did it again. This was no mistake.

Then his hands were down there, rubbing against my bottom as he slid down from the couch onto the floor. He flipped me over. I lay there motionless as his stinky tongue wagged in and out of my mouth.

It couldn't have been longer than a few minutes of making out with what must have felt like a mannequin. I had seen people kissing on the movies but it was nothing like this.

Darren was eighteen. I was twelve. It felt really wrong and completely uninvited. I excused myself abruptly from the floor, pulling his hand out of my pants, and headed for the kitchen.

He seemed to get the message and scampered off upstairs.

I opened the white balsa wood pantry door, shielding me from the living room. I mindlessly scanned its contents. I felt safe.

After a few more Darren incidents, I learned that I could protect myself by pulling my dresser in front of my bedroom door, which didn't have a lock on it. When the coast was clear, I crawled in bed with my mom. She sensed something was wrong. After days of her questions, I told her what happened, crying as if it was my fault. A police officer met with me at school and the problems with Darren ended.

However, going to the pantry didn't.

It was my M.O. I took up babysitting that summer, and pillaged other cabinets. I'd use my money I had earned to go the convenience store or ride my bicycle to the donut shop for a dozen. Once I fell and squished all the donuts, but ate them anyway. I had to use a spoon for the donut filling that sprayed out on the box.

My fingers grew deft at pulling confections out of packages without a single sound of the crinkling wrapper. I could hold food in my cheek like a hamster, masterfully chewing without making a sound. My mom would find piles of empty food wrappers under my bed. I stopped letting her clean my room.

I gained forty pounds that summer. When I returned to school, everybody seemed to know I tattled.

"Sexual harassment, stop, drop and roll," Donna and her friends would call out to me for the next year after they saw me. It didn't make any sense, but each time they shouted it out, it rang through me, making my eyes well and my stomach churn. I wanted to hide.

I walked around the middle school hallways with my shoulders slumped forward, head down, letting my long, greasy bangs cover my face.

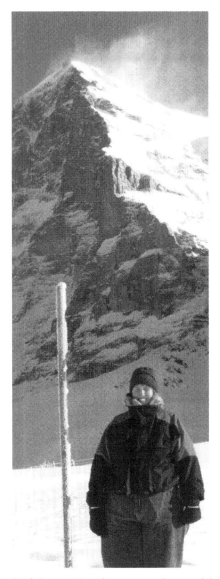

*Rock Bottom. It took a train and a gondola
to get me up this mountain in Switzerland.*

2. OVER THE HUMP

n high school, I started to get involved — from soccer to service clubs. I found a core group of friends—Bridget, Christie and Julia. But eating was still there for me to cope with everything—a good grade, a date rejection, or a bad day. By graduation, my weight was more than 250 pounds.

My friends and I all ended up going to the University of Vermont, where I relished the open meal plan. I grazed my way through the day and drank most nights. I didn't have a scale, but a visit to the doctor showed I topped 300 pounds by the end of freshman year.

I wasn't active, other than walking to class, parties and bars, but when someone suggested a daytime outing to Camel's Hump, it sounded exciting.

As a Vermont girl, it seemed only natural for me to join them. Sitting at the bottom of the mountain, I was humiliated that I did.

Five minutes up the trail, I thought my heart might explode. But I hunched over, yanked my sweat-soaked shorts from my flabby thighs and continued up the trail of Vermont's second highest peak, Camel's Hump.

My friends nudged me on, and then slowed to stay with me. But twenty minutes into the five-hour climb, my hyperventilating breath sounded like a fast-moving train. Everyone but my friend Christie had continued up the trail.

I told her, it was no use, I had to turn back. I was a University of Vermont freshman and my weight had caught up with me.

Christie looked relieved, but still asked, "Are you sure?"

I was. It wasn't safe for me to continue. She wished me well and headed up the mountain with sprite-like steps to catch up with the others. At nearly 300 pounds, I lumbered down to the trailhead.

I thought climbing Camel's Hump was a good idea. It was a beautiful summer day and I had hiked the same mountain, slowly, in middle school. But as my weight climbed it was harder to do most things. At the bottom of the mountain, I realized the only real walks I took those days were to class and to work. Sometimes I just slept in.

While I waited by the locked car, I dipped into my backpack loaded with a diet soda and bags upon bags of candy, including a pound of M&Ms (which I told myself I'd share). I made a sandwich. I brought an apple. I'm sure the goodies amounted to twice, maybe three times, the calories I would have burned on the whole hike.

I felt ashamed in the moments between shoving M&Ms in my mouth, by the handful. Sometimes I'd just tip my head back and pour them from the bag on to my tongue. I skipped the sandwich and apple in case my fellow hikers wanted to stop for lunch. I buried the empty wrappers in my backpack before my friends returned looking healthy, refreshed, energized. I looked like a lump on a log.

"How was it?" I asked. Before they answered, I launched into a barrage of excuses about why I had to stop: "I felt under-the-weather"; "I sprained my ankle two years ago and it's never been the same."

I knew why I couldn't climb Camel's Hump. My weight weighed me down like a wool coat that summer day. I worried my friends had talked about me all the way up and down the mountain. Maybe that was just me, beating myself up in my own mind: How could you let yourself get so fat, so lazy, and so pathetic?

I slunk my amorphous six-foot-tall body down in the car and headed back to campus feeling bloated and bigger than my half-dozen hiking friends combined.

Among my friends from high school who went to the University of Vermont with me, I was the happy-go-lucky heavy girl. I grew to be a great conversationalist as guys talked to me, trying to score with my girlfriends who shopped in the juniors section of clothing stores. Now I was solidly at my own plus-sized stores.

My first hookups were in the dark corners of fraternity houses and an under-the-radar relationship with a guy who slept with lots of girls, including one in the neighboring dorm room (I could hear them one night through the cinderblocks. He kept calling after that. I returned to him, thinking I couldn't get anyone better.)

I didn't score a boyfriend of my own until twenty-five-cent-draft night at a basement Irish pub. I had a pocket full of quarters. That night, after a good $2 worth of beer, my good friend Drew and I started flirting and then kissing.

Drew was a long-haired, potbelly fraternity brother who flunked out of the University of Vermont, twice. That night, when he lost his virginity, we started to date. He was a pure-hearted fellow, who immediately thought of me, and each person he met, as a friend. I always loved his eyes, cool blue pools of calm. I loved the lilt of Phish or Grateful Dead music that played while we sat smoking in his room, a dark air-conditioned vault on a hot summer day.

We made a weekend ritual of eating enough Chinese food for eight people and watching X-Files and The Simpsons re-run marathons. Our only regular activity was social drinking at his fraternity house or bars. He'd sleep until 2 p.m. and I would lie next to him, wondering when he'd get up instead of starting my day.

My friends worried he was sucking the ambition from my life, or at least giving me an excuse to sink. I didn't think about dumping him. I loved his sweetness. I loved that he accepted me, fat rolls and all. I loved that he was his own person, even if he was a little lost. Besides, I wondered who else in the world could love me.

When school was no longer an option for Drew, he became a ski instructor for the winter. In the summer, he was a camp counselor near the New Hampshire border, where he'd gone himself as a boy. I'd visit him during breaks between camp sessions. He pushed two cots together in his canvas-covered platform tent. It was an amazing place to make love after a rainstorm or on a soft, June evening.

What was even more amazing was that in a few short weeks of intimacy, we went from having sex in the dark, to candlelight, to daylight. I still covered myself with sheets between the action and slept wearing a t-shirt and underwear, but I never knew I could trust someone so much with my body, a body that even I hated.

But Drew was out of money. He decided to move to his mother's attic in Short Hills, New Jersey. I followed. I figured since we had just celebrated our one-year anniversary, this

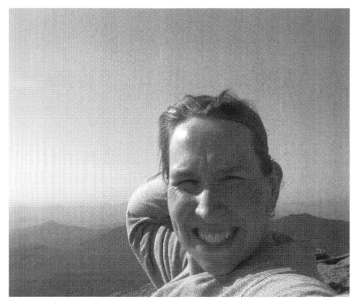

On top of Camel's Hump, Vermont's second highest peak.

relationship could be going somewhere. I imagined a wedding in a park. I'd hold a bunch of daisies and we'd cry during our vows.

With all my babysitting experience, I started to look for work as a live-in nanny. I figured that would take some of the pressure off my relationship with Drew, so we didn't have to live together right away. I could tell he felt crammed with me in his mother's house.

I came across an interesting listing. A family was looking for a nanny for their two boys with developmental disabilities. Joseph, nine, was autistic. David, seven, had ADHD. During the first interview, the straightforward father told me the challenges of the job including, "We're fat, and we're slobs."

Sounds perfect, I thought. I took the job.

A month after my move to my live-in job, Drew finally expressed concern for my weight, saying, "You must be so big in order to fit the size of your enormous heart."

That was how he broke up with me. I was mortified and dealt with it as I would any pain: I ate. I'd push snack cakes in my mouth-one after another. I'd finish a box of ten in one seating. My mouth felt slicked with trans fats. My stomach felt sick but I rarely stopped eating before the bottom of a box.

That next year, my weight peaked at about 360 pounds—I'm not exactly sure what the precise weight was since most scales stop at 350 and the needle was far above that.

I had to lie down to zip up my size 28 jeans, the highest size in many plus-sized clothing stores. My gut rolled over the belt line. I couldn't move. Even stairs were a challenge. I would grasp the railing and pull my way up.

I feared being bed-bound with a closet full of muumuus. I decided to start taking some action.

My weight dropped about thirty pounds because I started walking regularly, but rarely broke a sweat. I'd go to weight loss groups-even Overeaters Anonymous meetings-and swing by the drive-thru for a burger with fries on the way home.

Nothing stuck. The first batch of pounds, maybe 15 or so, came off without really trying. It was probably just water weight. After the initial thirty or so pounds were gone, losing weight was hard. Or maybe I made it hard. When I dropped weight, I was showered with attention. I would feel naked—exposed to the world.

People would say, "I can see it in your face."

I would look in the mirror, delighted with my progress. Somewhere inside I would get scared losing weight. I would find excuses to get off track such as a vacation or a bad day. Then

I'd gain again.Food had a way of consuming me. Call it compulsive overeating, food addiction, binging, a lack of willpower or whatever. When I was in a rut my hunger was insatiable. I went back to the cupboards and the refrigerator again and again looking for something, anything to fill the void. Of course, nothing did.

For a while I thought if I lost weight, Drew might want me back. It seemed like he did. I didn't know anyone else, so we continued to hang out, having a more off-than-on relationship for the next year or so.

Drew went from working in a game shop in the mall to being a waiter at chain restaurant. As a live-in nanny, I had lots of disposable income. I stocked his mini-fridge in the attic with fancy micro brews. I bought him a Star Trek phaser remote control.

His attic became a social club of sorts, an after-hours party for his bar outings.

It was in the attic that I met Drew's friend from around the block, Chris. Chris had just returned from five months in Central America and walked up the stairs with a scraggly traveler's beard. He brought a tapestry from Guatemala for Drew.

Drew immediately hung it on the ceiling, next to the other paisley cloths billowing under the breeze of his window-lodged air conditioner.

I immediately adored, maybe even envied Chris' adventurous spirit. He became an editor at a small market research company, and immediately became a part of the crew. After all, he and Drew had played Dungeons & Dragons together as teens. Chris was raised Quaker, learning an innate sense of accepting people for who they were. Of course, he was a bit of an oddball himself.

After Thursday night jogs, Chris came by Drew's attic to watch Friends and the rest of NBC's "Must See TV" line up. During ER's opening credits, Chris would get up and lunge forward with a punch along with Dr. Benton.

In August, I read a Star-Ledger article about an upcoming meteor shower. I brought up the idea of going outside to see it, at a scenic vista pullover off of Interstate 78. Drew passed. He was tired; besides, a new episode of the X-Files was playing that night. Chris was into it, so we went together on the hot summer night and watched falling stars on the hood of my car. I talked about Drew the whole time.

In an effort to get Drew motivated, his father, a Wall Street wizard, arranged for him to move to Hong Kong to learn the finance world from a good friend. Drew spent his energy elsewhere and met an Austrian woman who finally set him straight. Eventually, Drew even cut his hair.

When Drew left, I was busy being a full-time nanny, attending Montclair State University full-time to finish my degree, and working as managing editor for the student newspaper. Still, I made sure my Thursday night schedule was clear so Chris and I could continue our ritual of watching Friends. I loved how balanced Chris was and sought to meet his standards. Each time we met, one of us was responsible for picking up Boston Market, a somewhat healthy fast food, for dinner.

I cycled through a relationship with a fantastic kisser from Scotland who proposed marriage to stay in the United States longer, or at least legally. The answer was no.

Then, I had an odd yearlong every-night phone relationship with a roadie from one of my favorite bands. He sent me postcards from California, encouraging me to visit. When I got there, he didn't want me to let on to others that we had slept together. It was over.

But in the meantime I got a job—a great job—in California. The dot-com boom was in full swing and websites were hiring journalists for double or triple what they were making at a newspaper. So even though I had no experience, I booked a trip to do interviews, pitched story ideas, and even tried to crash a press conference. I got a gig at the biggest newspaper I applied for the Ventura County Star, with a circulation of nearly 100,000. Even without a West Coast love interest, I was going.

About a month before graduation, as I walked David, one of the boys I was a nanny for, home from school, I fell and felt a snap in my right foot. David wandered ahead and I couldn't walk. When David's father arrived home and my foot still throbbed, I called Chris.

I told Chris I didn't want to trouble him but thought maybe I should go to the hospital, being that I couldn't walk and all. He came right over, helped me get into his Mercury Sable wagon and drove straight to Boston Market so we could eat dinner before the long emergency room wait. He went in to the restaurant, picked up our dinner, and we ate in the front seat of his car. I didn't even have to tell him which sides I wanted, two servings of sweet potatoes.

At Saint Barnabas Hospital, a radiologist took images of my foot, which stung as I tried to align it along the white cross-marked board. When she returned to the room, I asked her what the news was. She said it wasn't good, but I'd have to wait to hear it officially from the doctor.

My fifth metatarsal, the bone along the outside of my right foot, had snapped. The doctor gave me a prescription for a

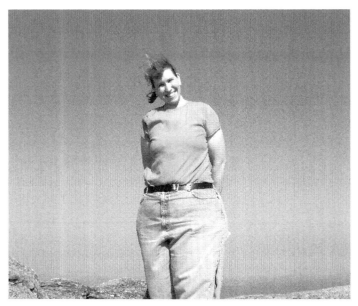

Standing proud on top of Camel's Hump to celebrate my 31st birthday.

painkiller and told me I'd be in a cast for six weeks. I came out to meet Chris in the hospital's lobby with a frown and crutches.

"Oh, no," he said.

"Yup, it's broken."

He pulled the car around to the entrance. On the way home, Chris stopped at Haagen-Dazs for ice cream. I was in love.

The trouble was it was two months before my move to California to take my first job as a journalist. After a few drinks at my going away party, we found ourselves kissing all night long. We decided to give our relationship a try from a distance.

We had long-distance dates. I would watch the early showing of a movie in California and he would catch the late show in New Jersey, then we would call each other and talk about it. Frequent flier miles and minute overages aside, it wasn't a sure thing.

During Chris's first visit to California, we walked along the boardwalk in Venice Beach, passing an assortment of beautiful-bikini clad women, tattoo-covered guys and a few folks who seemed stuck in the 1960s. I reached for his hand. He didn't take mine.

That night, instead of folding myself into Chris' arms, I pulled myself to the edge of the mattress. I stared at the dust bunnies, trying to come up with the words for the conversation I didn't want to have. "What's going on here?"

Chris wasn't sure he wanted to stay together. We danced around reasons why our relationship wouldn't work. Maybe it was the weight. Maybe it was the distance.

Back and forth, we struggled with breaking up or continuing on. Somewhere in the hours of conversation, the only thing we were sure of was that we couldn't imagine not being in each other's lives and "just friends" wouldn't do.

The next day we went to Paradise Cove, a restaurant along a secluded stretch of the Pacific Ocean. We shared a pan of paella and decided to walk along the private beach. We held hands.

After a year in California, watching Friends in different time zones and thousands of frequent flier miles, I moved back to New Jersey. Chris proposed three years later.

I was sure that he would back out of the wedding at the last minute. I was afraid he would have a Shallow Hal moment and realize how big I really was. He didn't; he took me for fatter and for thinner.

For the most part, my weight didn't seem to bother Chris. He only seemed disappointed when I set out to lose weight, only to give in to temptation. I could feel his glance when I reached for seconds and he knew I was out of Weight Watchers Points, calories or carbs. He didn't have to say anything. I felt bad enough, but I overate anyway.

My weight never matched Chris' somewhat-slim figure. He'd run. I'd walk. He'd have breakfast, lunch, and dinner. I'd graze in meal-sized portions all day long even though I told people I was on a diet.

I was stuck in a constant yo-yo between 300 and 335 pounds. I thought I wanted to lose weight but seemed scared of the consequences. What would I do without my security blanket that had comforted me for so long?

For a long time, fat had been my insulation against so many bad things-my parents' divorce at age nine, a sexual assault at age twelve by my cousin's eighteen-year-old friend, and being the "pretty face" who couldn't get a prom date. It even made me numb to the embarrassing moments of being overweight, like little girls asking if there was a baby in my tummy. No, I wasn't pregnant, but I was thirty and married. Motherhood, when time is no longer yours alone, was on the horizon. Even if I survived life in the morbidly obese column, my "to-do" list was getting longer and my time to complete my ambitions was getting shorter.

I started to look back at my life, especially at the failed Camel's Hump hike, and realized instead of cushioning me, fat was swallowing my dreams.

I often settled for standing in the lonely, cold comfort of an open refrigerator, searching for something to saturate what I was feeling at a given moment: happy, sad, fearful, frustrated, anything. I didn't need bread. I would eat peanut butter right from the jar. I'd eat anything to feel nothing.

I wore all black because that was supposed to appear slimming. I hated trying to look pretty but feeling ugly. I hated that my pants wore out in the crotch from the friction between my thighs, and that at any minute the seam on my seat could burst open.

I felt like a hundred-pound anvil was chained around my waist when I climbed stairs. Once I "jogged" a 5K, and Chris, who was running the 10K, finished before I did. I hated feeling out-of-breath after only a few minutes of playing basketball together.

I was an armchair adventurer, pining over glossy Mountain Travel Sobek adventure catalogues offering tours up Mont Blanc, Everest, Kilimanjaro, and Machu Picchu-right before polishing off a king-sized Kit-Kat bar. I used to tell myself I would love to do a hike like that when I lost weight.

But I hadn't lost the weight. If I continued the way I was going, I never would. I didn't want to regret not living fully while I was young and healthy.

I longed to be one of those Nalgene bottle-toting girls. The healthy, fleece-wearing granola-chic gal with good skin. But I wasn't.

On New Year's 2005, I found myself in a familiar ritual, on a diet and about to write a resolution about how much weight I wanted to lose. I was down to 286 pounds, the lowest I had been in a decade and I wanted to keep up the momentum. Writing down "I will lose forty pounds this year" on past New Year's never got me anywhere. I needed to get going.

I thought about what I wanted to do. I thought about how weight was holding me back. I thought about Camel's Hump. I decided: Mountain climbing was my new mission. But Camel's Hump was just a day hike, the kind of thing most people pack a picnic lunch for and do in an afternoon. I wanted a bigger goal, something to really get me moving.

I had been interested in the Grand Canyon since Steve, my Star-Ledger bureau chief—a nature photographer who wears "Life is Good" T-shirts when he's not working—showed me pictures of his trip there. I remembered thinking, I want to go too.

I wanted to go but was afraid I had become the kind of tourist who pulled up in a car to the ledge of a scenic vista, parked as close as possible, and took a quick look. I was afraid of getting there, then leaving quietly, disappointed in myself, certain to binge away my feelings.

So there it was, my 2005 resolution:

Hike down (and more importantly back up) the Grand Canyon.

I booked a late-September backcountry permit as a bold move, assuming that I would be physically fit enough to tackle the trip down a steep switchback trail to the Colorado River and back up the following day. It would take a lot of work to get there.

The Grand Canyon Bright Angel Trail would be an unforgiving ten-mile uphill, 4,100-foot climb. As soon as we registered to hike it, the National Parks Service sent a DVD complete with dramatizations of people slumping over from heat exhaustion and a first-person account of someone who set a hillside ablaze after burning toilet paper.

The DVD warned that park rangers are not "legally responsible" to rescue you, and for good reason. Every year, people die there. More often than not, it's because they were unprepared.

I didn't want to be left for dead, nor the subject of the next public service announcement saying fat women shouldn't attempt the Grand Canyon. I might not be super slim by the time I got there, but I could be prepared. If I were going to have the strength to conquer the Grand Canyon that September, I figured I'd first have to get over the measly 2,600 feet of Camel's Hump.

I filled my calendar with workouts and started spending five days a week in the gym. I sweated through hours on the treadmill, spinning classes, and yoga classes. I would run up and down the staircase at the gym again and again and again.

On weekends, Chris and I hiked. It had been a decade since I let my hiking boots get dirty, sinking slightly in the mud, collecting crusty leaves in the laces. My boots were stiff, having only been for short walks through the snow, and I was sure a blister was burning through my heel.

I waddled at a nearly-300-pound-woman pace behind Chris.

"Baby, wait up," I'd say as he bolted ahead of me at Jockey Hollow, a former Revolutionary War encampment, now a National Park in Harding, New Jersey. Even though the trail turned and he walked out of sight, I could hear the corn flake-crunch of dead leaves under his boots.

As I trudged through Jockey Hollow on an early-March day, I worried that I had dragged Chris into another doomed weight loss attempt, the kind he'd suffer through for weeks, even though I had secretly stopped by the middle of the first day.

If I was going to have the strength to hike the Grand Canyon in six months, I needed to get going.

We started with flatter ventures. I let my feet remember the natural roll of the earth under hiking boots. Even the easiest trails felt strenuous at first. Chris would roam ahead and then double back, tapping his thigh as if to say, "Here, girl."

It irked me, but I wanted to catch up. Instead of expending

energy yelling at him, I focused on moving stronger and faster.

The first puny hills of Jockey Hollow left me with measured breath. I tried not to talk so Chris didn't know how out-of-shape I was on these beginner trails. I hoped my flushed cheeks would be mistaken for wind burn. The day was still.

In the midst of self-doubt, I heard my yoga instructor Reina's voice in my head, "You have to start somewhere or you're nowhere." Reina was a loving Jewish earth mother, who cheered me on this new path of hiking for health. In her classes, I'd soak in her messages of self-love and gratitude.

After the Jockey Hollow jaunt, and from then on, I developed a ritual of post-hike stretching with a sun salutation, a series of forward bends and lunges, in which I'd thank the mountain for being strong under my feet and my feet for being strong on the mountain.

After a couple of hikes, I was the one pushing forward our training schedule. I picked trails with higher and higher elevations. First was Mount Philo in Vermont-a 650-foot hill. Then, I conquered Mount Tammany, a 1,200-foot climb along the Delaware River in New Jersey.

The more I climbed, the stronger I became, and the more weight I lost. By June, I had dropped thirty-one pounds to 255 pounds. It was the lowest weight I'd been since high school.

I decided my life would be filled with new celebrations, new ways of living. For my thirty-first birthday, I would conquer Camel's Hump.

I was up at daybreak, a soft pink sky framed by the Green Mountains. I pulled on jeans that had fit me snugly a few short weeks ago, but now had to be held up by a belt. My daypack had already been loaded with trail mix, fruit, and water.

I couldn't find anyone to go with me: my husband and

friends all had other commitments. In a way, I was grateful: What if I didn't make it up? Then, there would be no one who would know.

Once I stepped on the trail, the maple canopy enclosed me. Camel's Hump's earthy aroma was so familiar and made me think of my attempt a decade before. I worried that this journey would end like the last one, still so vivid in my mind. If it did, I hoped it would happen fast before I ran into other hikers.

I was alone in the early hours of the climb. My steps were sure, steady and strong. When I walked, I could hear my breath—heavy but controlled—and the crunch of leaves under boot. When I stopped to rest, the rustling breeze overhead beckoned me toward the peak.

I grew more tired as the trail grew steeper. My feet became clumsy, nearly tripping over the rocks. I found myself angry that I had let myself go for so long. I was still obese by any standard.

I found myself at a plateau junction, where I could see the summit, reaching up like the hump of a camel. It's the face of many Vermont postcards, one that teased me since my last defeat. I would only need to walk one more mile to get there.

I scrambled over rocks and came uncomfortably close to the ledge on sections of trail, but kept going up until there was nowhere else to climb. As I reached the summit, the view left me breathless. This is what I had been missing, a top-of-the-world feeling of accomplishment.

A mother, her daughter, and their dog had passed me on the way up. I found them there at the summit. I asked them to take my picture. The mother told me she hikes the Camel's Hump trail almost every morning.

I told her that was impressive, as it had taken me ten years to climb this mountain.

3. GRAND CANYON

The first time I saw the Grand Canyon was the afternoon before I hiked it. We drove north from an eggs Benedict breakfast with our friends in Phoenix, Arizona. It was hot, over 90 degrees, but it's what we expected for a late-September day in the desert. After a few, "Hey, look at that cactus" comments, I got to thinking, What's the big deal with the Grand Canyon? Even Williams, Arizona, where we stopped a few miles from the ridge for lunch, felt like a movie set town. It didn't give the feeling of what was to come.

The northbound road made a distinct turn to the left. We flashed our National Parks Pass and, a few speed bumps later, the bottom dropped out of world to the right of our rental car. The endless range of red rocks, stretching up from the Colorado River thousands of feet below, made me scared to even get out of the vehicle. But eventually, I did.

That afternoon before our hike, I sauntered to the right of the path, as far from the edge as I could, to a railed lookout. I chose a spot close enough to the ridge for my knees to wobble.

I looked down below at the Tonto Plateau. It was so far down that the trail looked like dental floss pulled through the sand. I saw ant-like hikers making their way across the plateau and then drop out of sight.

I had worried that even though the Grand Canyon was billed as a seemingly endless series of switchbacks, that I would somehow land in an El Capitan rock climbing moment, gripping with all my might to lift myself to safety, but then slip to my death. My friends and family would say, "If she had only lost more weight."

It wasn't my imagination. The Grand Canyon can be a dangerous place.

Unlike a typical mountain, the hardest part comes last, when most climbers take twice as long to go back up the canyon as compared to the time it takes to go down. It's so hot that sweat evaporates instantly. The dry air made my tongue feel like a pumice stone. The guidebooks instructed Chris and me to drink enough water to make our pee turn clear. The Lonely Planet Grand Canyon National Park guide called the South Kaibab trail "steep, rough and wholly exposed" with a dearth of shade and water.

We would each have to carry three liters of water to drink on the way down, praying that the water supplies would be working along the Bright Angel Trail, on our way up, when we needed it most.

Our preparedness for this trek would rival the Boy Scouts. We followed every National Park Service restriction to the letter. I previously signed up for backcountry pass (an envelope-sized tag to attach to my backpack) precisely on the earliest date we could. Thousands of people apply for them, but only hundreds are issued. We got our second choice of routes, the South Rim loop-South Kaibab down and Bright Angel up. We had wanted to do a rim-to-rim hike, requiring a van to backtrack from one end to the other when we finished the adventure. Nevertheless, the South Rim loop route was a fine choice and would allow us to fit in some sightseeing in Utah once we finished the canyon climb.

I booked a humble room with a shared bathroom at the Bright Angel Lodge, and a fancy dinner at El Tovar, a historic lodge within the national park, on the South Rim. At El Tovar, I ordered the duck, normally a bit fattier than I would have chosen, but I decided that I needed energy for the days ahead. For a brief moment, I thought it could be my last meal.

That night, after I checked and double checked my backpack, Chris drifted off to sleep. I got out of bed several times to pee in the common bathroom down the hall. I tried to be quiet, hoping not to awaken other adventurers. If they had planned to do the same hike we were, they would need the rest.

~~~

"Can you run the Boston Marathon?"

That was the first line of a warning sign we saw as we approached the South Kaibab trailhead. Uh, no, I thought. I took every staircase possible in the months before our Grand Canyon trek. The first two hours of each morning were spent at the gym, walking on an ever-escalating treadmill, pounding up a moving staircase, or sweating my way through a spinning class. But a marathon? No.

It was about 6 a.m. A soft pink hue remained in the late-fall sky, and a public service announcement was telling me I could very likely die on this jaunt down the canyon. I read the rest of the sign about a woman who ran the Boston Marathon but was ill-prepared when it came to the Grand Canyon. She hiked sixteen miles carrying an energy bar, an apple, and a sixteen-ounce bottle of water with her. She died of dehydration and heat exhaustion.

We didn't need to carry all of our food, as I had arranged a hikers' stew dinner and pre-dawn pancakes, eggs, and sausage breakfast at the Phantom Ranch camp at the bottom of the canyon. Still, my backpack, which nearly pulled me to the ground, was stuffed with fixings for a crab cake lunch. I had a half-dozen bagels with as many individual peanut butter and jelly containers (swiped from restaurants sporadically in the months before). I had three pounds of Trader Joe's trail mix and four Luna Bars. We each carried three liters of water at all times, just like we did when we were training.

If I were to perish in the Grand Canyon, it wouldn't have been due to a lack of food and water.

Perhaps I went a little overboard. But I was going by the Parks Service advice, "The dietary needs of a Grand Canyon hiker are similar to those of a runner in a marathon."

For the last few months of training, I had taken on Oprah's Boot Camp. I needed something serious. This plan had eight workouts a week (of course, there's only seven days a week). On this plan, I had to work out twice two times a week, and got one rest day.

But even more dramatically, I abstained from all refined sugar, which led to some interesting moments, such as nearly spilling into a tearful tantrum when a caffeine-free soda tumbled out of the vending machine. I had pushed the button for a fully-loaded one. Caffeine was my only vice left.

I didn't have another dollar to get the real thing from the other machine down the hall. My coworker Greg let me borrow a dollar. Greg and my newspaper colleagues who sat near me were all supportive of me, listening to the incessant whining about what I could and could not eat.

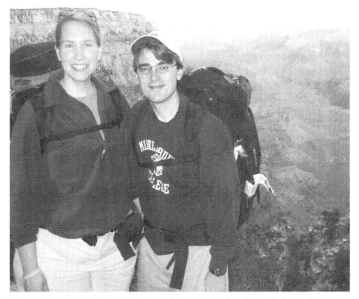

Starting our way down the Grand Canyon's South Kaibab trail.

"Not even sushi? Oh yeah, white rice."

I was hoping to drop forty pounds, the weight of my backpack. I dropped twenty. Of course, I worried it wouldn't be enough, but I felt strong, steady, and ready.

The first few steps of the South Kaibab Trail felt like stepping off the end of the earth. The skinny switchbacks hugged close to the edge. At times I worried my still-bulging hips would tilt my body weight over the side.

Vertigo can easily set in walking down the side of a canyon, with a 4,000 foot drop on the edge. Every once in a while I couldn't help but glance and felt a kaleidoscope tilt of woozy staring into the crevasse below. I returned my gaze to the wall, steadying my vision and my mind. I thought, Don't look down.

The momentum carried me down the canyon, but carefully

so. I walked in measured galumphs, sometimes taking one step at a time, to be sure both feet landed on solid ground. I thought about little other than my rhythm.

About a mile into the descent, we came across a beautiful platform. Chris wandered to its edge and rested his backpack against the rock. I paused to see the morning light setting the rocks around him aglow. This canyon seemed like it was ours. The view was better than a postcard, it was alive. I was alive, and really, truly living.

Less than ten percent of the people who visit the Grand Canyon travel its backcountry trails to the bottom. Now, because of my hard work, I would be one of them.

There is a point in every hike when I wonder who could have possibly come up with such a crazy plan (that point came a few minutes into this hike). Why can't I be a "girly girl" who flutters at the thought of mosquitoes and squirms knowing that you're camping at the same level as snakes—poisonous rattling snakes?

Then I remembered. I'm not a girly girl.

Now that I was over the excuses for not living my life, I lived for this stuff. I loved being able to describe places most people don't go or coming across someone who has hiked the same perilous path as I had, reveling about how hard it was, knowing we each accomplished something great.

I loved the awe, the absolute awe of seeing a 4,000-feet drop, and realizing that soon enough, step by step, I'd be there too (safely). So down, down, down we went. Each plateau exposed another set of ledges that we would have to traverse in endless switchbacks carved into the side of the cliff.

Most times my feet were sure. Sometimes, I felt tired and stumbled. But on and on we went through the red rocks, surrounded by big, blue sky. As the people passed on mule backs, I would know that I did this on my own two feet.

We found our way through ten miles of knee-jarring descent, over the Colorado River and to Bright Angel Campground. We set up our tent and made crab cakes served on bagels. They were a little dry, but a welcome feast after the hard work. After a park ranger lecture about bats later that night, we headed back to our tent under a blanket of stars.

~~~

Our ascent would begin at 5 a.m. to beat the heat. A good pace would be a mile an hour. The trail is ten miles long.

As per the ranger's instruction, we stopped every hour. We rested, we took our over-stuffed backpacks off and lay back on the ground, feet straight up in the air.

It was a way to rest and release your legs. I wasn't sure what the science was behind the suggestion, I was just grateful for a chance to rest every hour and eat trail mix.

The three liters of water on my back didn't seem like a lot to carry considering how much weight I had on me before this portion of the journey.

The journey back up to the top of the Grand Canyon's South Rim involves traversing the zigzag switchbacks. We had been at it for eight hours when suddenly, it felt very, very hard. It was hardest we had ever hiked, but we had a system. Hike, rest, and then move on. Having a prescribed way of getting up the ledge worked, instead of me tagging behind Chris all the time or him rushing to the top. We were told to rest and we did so.

The last mile, Chris was my rock, encouraging me to rest,

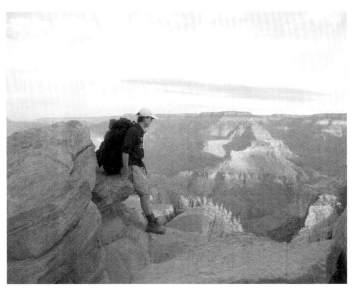

The amazing view of my husband and the Grand Canyon on the South Kaibab Trail.

drink, and then push on. During the last mile, which took close to two hours, it seemed like we stopped and rested every few steps.

But then we got to the ledge, back on solid ground. We celebrated by sitting and enjoying the view with peanut butter and jelly sandwiches. We had done it—all the way down and back up again.

I was exhausted but felt fantastic. After a quick, smelly trip through the gift shop, we drove straight to Zion National Park.

We spent the evening in the hot tub of the Desert Pearl hotel in Springdale, Utah. Even if I wasn't close to wearing a bikini, I was proud of my new, smaller bathing suit. I could see pride as Chris looked at me.

We started our day in Zion with hot stone massages, booked

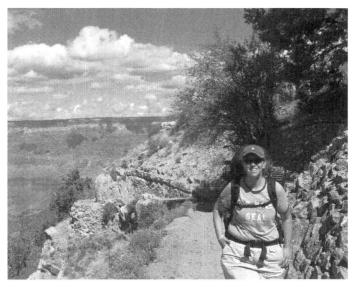

Ten miles of up, making my way up the Grand Canyon.

to celebrate our Grand Canyon climb. Relaxed but restless, we took out the Zion National Park trail map to figure out what to do next.

This could have been a day of "thank-God-I-made-it-out-of-bed" aches, made for a short, stretch-your-legs jaunt along the pretty Emerald Pools trail.

Instead, I picked Observation Point, the longest, hardest day hike on the map, a steep eight-mile trip that would take five hours round trip. It was the last listing in the "Strenuous" hike section. This was what amazed Chris the most—my newfound heart-pounding devotion to being healthy and strong. It was for me. But it was for him, too. Even though I was left with bulging calves and a few varicose spider veins from tugging around so much weight, I loved the way Chris looked at me.

The next day on the Observation Point trail, I squinted up

at the bright blue sky, a beautiful contrast to the chiseled Navajo soapstone trail on which we were standing. After I took a big swig from my half-empty Nalgene bottle, my eyes drifted down to find my husband's gaze upon me.

"You're like a different woman," Chris said. Perhaps my squinting eyes came across as a "What-on-earth-are-you-talking-about?" look. He continued, "No, really, think about it. You are so strong. You have such a sense of adventure now-more than before."

If I weren't already flushed from the two hours uphill through the wavy peach stones in Zion National Park, I would have blushed. Chris wasn't the type to shower me with affection and saccharine compliments. So to hear this, an hour before the apex of our hike, left me more breathless than the trail itself.

I put my hands on the fleece tied around my waist and sunk my hands on my hip bone. Since I had lost a total of 110 pounds from my top weight of more than 350 pounds, I had a new, strange fascination with my hip bone. I could finally feel its rock-hard edge rising above the waistband of my saggy jean shorts.

I especially loved the way Chris looked at me at that moment on Zion. There was an hour to Observation Point, but basking in Chris's admiration I felt even more determined.

The sip of water barely quenched my thirst and the arid climate made my tongue feel like a pumice stone, but I dropped a big, not-so-wet kiss on him. We embraced for a moment, trying not to wobble over the side of the trail before pressing on to the top.

The next day, we headed to Bryce Canyon and hit its longest trail, Fairyland Loop—eight miles, five hours by his side.

4. UPS AND DOWNS

I t was hard for people not to notice my weight loss. My pants draped like curtains on my belt. I swam in my shirts. By November 2005, I had conquered Camel's Hump and the Grand Canyon. My body felt strong, tight. I'd take two stairs at a time. Every once in a while, I felt a strange compulsion to lunge into warrior pose, a standing yoga position, with legs wide and arms outstretched, one in front and one in back, with a gaze over the front fingers.

But instead of keeping track of my adventures, most people kept tabs on how many pounds I had lost. The total: A little more than one hundred pounds.

My friend and managing editor Marilyn would ask me weekly how much weight I had lost and tell me how great I'd look, even on weeks when I gained three pounds. It was the same with a forty-something advertising representative. I didn't even know her name, but she asked me about my weight each time we passed in the hallway or ran into each other in the ladies' room. This would always be followed by her lamenting about her own weight loss woes. I always thought she looked quite fit, if not skinny.

For someone who shielded herself from attention with extra weight in the past, this could be downright intimidating. It was like a spotlight that followed me. At work, people even called me "skinny" when I passed. Mostly, people wanted to know:

"How did you do it?"

"How long did it take you?"

"What did you eat?"

Some people danced around the topic of "the surgery." They'd tell me about friends they knew who had bariatric surgery, a procedure that limits the size of the stomach, giving patients less room to eat, helping them lose dozens, if not hundreds, of pounds. Then, they would casually ask if I had the same thing done.

"Eating less, moving more," was my smug answer, but it worked when I was in a hurry. Besides, most people lost interest in the conversation when I said it had taken years to lose the weight.

People wanted the answer in a neat little package, an instant diet plan. I knew that if I endorsed a particular diet plan, the next day half of my office would have signed up for the same program.

But my weight loss wasn't an all-in-one shot. It took a lot of little plans. It took Weight Watchers here, Oprah's Boot Camp there, South Beach bars from time to time, a 4 p.m. ritual of eating Luna Bars, and working out (a lot) to get rid of one hundred pounds. I had to find out what worked for me. Sometimes nothing did.

Sometimes life got cloudy, with no time to shop for healthy food, to whip up a low-calorie meal, or to pack a baggie of mini-carrots and a diet soda in my work bag. Sometimes, an emotional whirlwind touched down and I'd eat. I'd eat a lot. I wanted a big bacon cheeseburger and large fries. I needed a big bacon cheeseburger and large fries.

There's more to losing weight than before and after pictures. I hated this notion that just because I was on a diet, if I didn't to get down to my goal weight, then I failed. Wasn't losing ten or twenty pounds at a stretch moving forward? My weight crept up in spurts; why couldn't I lose it in the same way?

~~~

Chris and I sat together in my in-laws' attic. We were living with his parents in Short Hills, New Jersey, to save money. Neither of us had jobs after he finished graduate school, and we were a few months from getting married.

After Chris graduated from the University of Michigan Business School (earning a Masters in Business Administration, with distinction), we decided to take a break, a round-the-world trip. We booked a journey starting in Brazil for a friend's wedding, and added stops in Thailand, India, and Europe. It would be our $50-a-day pre-honeymoon adventure. We figured we could always make more money, but never make more time.

When we returned to the United States, Chris' resume had stopped circulating through companies. He had to start his job search over again, resumé after unanswered resumé. He got lots of interviews but no immediate job offers.

Before I left on the trip, I was promised my old job back at the Courier News, a newspaper serving Central Jersey where I had worked before moving to Michigan. When I called my editor in late July, I learned he'd have to wait for a hiring freeze to thaw out before he could bring me back on staff.

Chris and I spent the unemployed hours wedding planning and job searching. We took turns on the computer in the attic. Between me, Chris, his gracious parents, Robin and Jim, the computer was in demand, an almost Grand Central Station. I was waiting for my turn to check e-mail, hoping for one from the Courier News, telling me it was time to start work.

Chris wrapped up his online job search for the day and had uploaded the photos from our round-the-world trip. We were going to send an e-mail blast of photos to our friends, knowing only a few people would click through them.

As a heavy woman, I avoided the camera as much as possible. My husband caught me in a few shots. One photo from Sylt, Germany showed me lagging behind on a beach walk. I looked exhausted even though the path was flat.

Chris turned to me with an otherwise innocent question: "Most people have a weight ceiling where they don't let their weight soar past a certain point. How come you never had one?"

It was one of those guy questions, the ones they ask and are so clueless that it could sting. I didn't even have a response because I didn't know the answer.

My weight had been above 300 pounds almost my entire adult life. Why was Chris asking this now? Perhaps it was the hundreds of trip photos that we were about to share with our friends. Perhaps he saw me as a fat person in those images, especially the ones from Thailand, where he and I became keenly aware of how big I was.

Most of the female tourists in Thailand were the sort out of the movie The Beach, wandering around in a bikini top and a batik cloth on the bottom. It was hard for me to find a wrap big enough to tie around my waist. I was ashamed trying them on in front of the vendors.

Staring isn't taboo in Thailand and laughter is a sign that someone is uncomfortable. On almost every corner in Thailand, tuk-tuk drivers stared and laughed at my huge body. Vendors did the same.

In Bangkok, a Vogel Tailors salesman took my measurements, in case I ever decided to order a custom-made suit. He wrote the numbers in a ledger, and read them out loud, first snickering and then dissolving into utter laughter. I was infuriated, and I told him that I would never buy a suit from him. It didn't seem to matter to the guy with the measuring tape around his neck: he was having too much fun making fun of me. Chris was stuck with his set of suits that he ordered the day before. They had already charged his credit card, and besides, it was a good deal for custom-made suits.

On the Thai island of Ko Phag Nan, the most humiliating incident was when we returned from the island of Ko Phag Nan to Ko Samui by ferry. The boat pulled to the dock, which seemed like it was wagging in time with the sea. It had that movie look to it—the kind that collapses underfoot when a hero runs across it. (Surely that hero wouldn't weigh the 300-plus pounds that I did at the time.) But as I drew closer to the front of the line, I recognized that wasn't the worst of it. To get from the boat to the dock, one had to cross a plank. This was no ordinary piece of wood. It was sun-weathered gray and had cracks in all sorts of spots along the grain.

When the receiving dock workers saw me in line, they spoke the international language of "Gulp!" There were two people boat side, helping people across. While every other passenger walked across carrying their backpacks, there seemed to be a sigh of collective relief when I thought to take mine off. Still, they looked scared that I wouldn't make the six-foot plank walk.

I let everyone, including my poor, patient husband, cross in front of me. Chris walked ahead of me because he didn't want to share the wood with my weight. He was already afraid of his own normal-size body bearing down on the creaking boards.

With a heave-ho, the boat crew helped me step on the plank. It couldn't have been more than a foot wide. After being the laughing stock of the Vogel Tailors, I knew I was well wider than that.

Many of the Thai island shores are shallow. That's why the ferry had to stop so far from the beach. I knew that if the wood gave way, I wouldn't be swallowed by the sea. I would come to a crashing death on the ocean's sandy bottom. *Forget diabetes, heart disease, or cancer from a decade of morbid obesity,* I thought, *weight would kill me this way.*

The ferry crew members' thin hands pushed under my ham-hock arms, to lift me up and make me as light as possible. I was on my own for a few steps and the wood bowed to my weight. The men on the other side reached out, almost to say "easy, easy" with beads of sweat and a look of strain on their faces.

My foot plunked down on the dock. My heart started beating again and I hurried along the dock, afraid to put pressure on any one board. I got to the shore and looked back to see all four of the men bowed down in laughter.

Seriously, how did I get so big? Why didn't it bother me?

I had stopped noticing myself. At my largest, I was clumsy, forgetting where my body began and ended, knocking over picture frames as I walked past end tables. For me, obesity was a strange, unspoken thing. I lost sight of what I had done to my own body. It was a secret that everyone could see. Typically, I tossed photos that showed my full girth. My friends took, or only showed me, photos from the waist up of my pear-shaped body.

I never owned full-length mirrors. I wore the top size at most plus stores, 28, even when I was at least fifty pounds too heavy for it. I couldn't admit that I had ballooned past the plus-sized clothing line into a bigger size range. I'd have to order clothing from the kind of catalogue that sold muumuus. I had to buy new clothes. I had to buy a size 32 pair of jeans. During a trip to Switzerland, when I had to take trains in order to get to the top of mountains, turtlenecks bunched up at my waist, because they were too tight to fit around my huge hips.

I left my in-laws' attic, went to our room (his parents' guest room), and opened up an empty page in my day planner, the kind of place where I would normally plot out my weight loss intentions. I started by numbering the axis with my weight, starting at my highest, which I guessed to be about 360 pounds, and numbering down to 130 pounds. Then I marked my age starting at age twelve, the year I was molested and gained forty pounds, and continued to my current age, thirty.

As best I could, I plotted out the path of my gain. For me, the last decade was pretty easy. I had been a serial dieter. I kept log upon log of weekly weigh-ins. I filled in the blanks with jaw-dropping memories of being on the scale. Some of it was guessing, a vague recollection of being the biggest, fattest person in my gym class.

My chart looked something like the Dow Jones Industrial Average during the Internet boom. There were little dips along the way, but my weight climbed steadily from age twelve to twenty-two. I tried to understand the connection between possibly related events and the numbers. Under each age, I wrote down a significant event in my life.

It started to spike as a young child as my parents were divorcing and then again when I was molested. I wrote "Lonely" from ages fourteen to sixteen when my weight went from 200 to 240 pounds. "Friends, hockey games" I wrote under ages

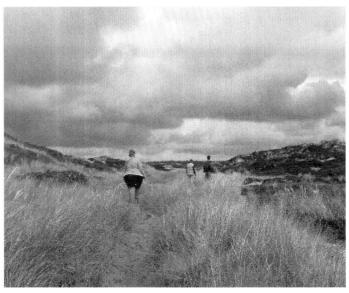

Lagging behind on a beach walk in Sylt, Germany.

sixteen to eighteen. My weight leveled out a bit, to about 250 pounds, during those years when I found a crew of good friends. We'd all go to the University of Vermont hockey games. I also played sports in high school, though I was never any good at them.

I marked age nineteen with "Greenwich, Connecticut." My weight climbed to about 260. I was a nanny there for about six months and discovered Monte Cristos, a deep-fried ham and cheese sandwich that is dusted with powdered sugar and dipped in raspberry jam. Even though I was underage, I learned how to get the waiter to bring me drink specials at the local restaurant. (For some reason, they never carded me.)

"Started dating Drew" marked the passage above 300 pounds, age twenty-one. My weight surged from there until about a year after our breakup. I marked the peak at 360, at age twenty-three.

Sometimes I couldn't think of an explanation for a weight loss or gain, other than I had fallen into a routine of eating far beyond my needs.

Then, there was a steady long term decline-like the stock market when reality burst the bubble-as I started to exercise and pay attention to my food intake. Even then, my weight went up and down over shorter periods. The chart looked a little like a mountain range.

I wished I had a cap on my weight, or some kind of warning like a pair of pants that felt too snug so I would lay off the ice cream. Why couldn't I be one of those people who feel fat when they're only pushing twenty pounds beyond their ideal weight range?

Since I started coating myself with weight as a young girl, I had no idea what my body would look or feel like as a thin person. All I knew how to do was be fat.

.

5. MOVING MOUNTAINS

After my hiking accomplishments, my weight sat at about 250 pounds. I felt pretty good about it, for a little while anyway. I thought I looked pretty good at 250 pounds. I could wear tops from normal-sized clothing stores. I had to have the bigger clothes I still liked tailored to fit me (though I had bagged up most of rest and donated them to charity).

People opened doors for me. They smiled back. People at the gym, whom I'd never met, would come over to my treadmill just to say, "You look great. Keep up the good work."

The random compliments continued long after my Grand Canyon glow wore off. Though since I wasn't training for anything, my trips to the gym started to feel purposeless.

My workouts slipped from sixty minutes on the stair stepper to forty-five minutes on the treadmill to the twenty-eight-minute fat burning cycle on the elliptical trainer without punching up the resistance one bit. I still did spinning, but after a year of the indoor stationary bicycle class, I could have done it in my sleep (particularly when I didn't crank up the resistance knob). I stopped weight resistance training all together. Some weeks, I only did yoga.

The less I exercised, the more I ate. I had opened an eating stop-gap and started to indulge again. Anything that was off-limits while in training—giant chocolate chip cookies at the checkout line, chips with an otherwise healthy Subway sub—started creeping into my lunch. I wondered if people noticed the fries in my Wendy's bag and whispered, "She's back on the sauce."

As I felt myself pulled into lethargy, almost a post-accomplishment depression, I knew I was the only one who would could get myself out of it. I also knew the longer I waited, the harder it would be.

I had climbed Camel's Hump. I had pushed myself to finish the ten-mile uphill Bright Angel Trail in the Grand Canyon. I didn't want to lose all I had worked for. I had to start thinking about what was next.

Around New Year's 2006, I decided to revisit my adventure catalogues and travel websites for inspiration. I clicked my way through countries I had never been, and kept coming across Mount Kilimanjaro, Africa's highest peak.

Located in Tanzania, it is one of the world's Seven Summits-the collection of tallest peaks from each continent. It is the world's tallest freestanding mountain, and I wanted to conquer it.

One website boasted Kilimanjaro as the highest mountain one could climb without supplemental oxygen, ice axes, and the like. Another said you could just walk to the top. The venture seemed exciting, exotic, and do-able. Plus, it could help keep my weight on a downward track.

The more I looked for trips, the more I found people using Kilimanjaro climbs as fund raisers. Climbers sought donations for their favorite charities on behalf of their monumental goal. There were plenty of causes to choose from: breast cancer, diabetes, cerebral palsy, and more.

This seemed like a brilliant idea. My weight loss could be for a good cause, turning all that attention (that sometimes I relished, sometimes I shied away from) and focusing it on something important. My workouts would have purpose again.

I decided that if Chris and I were to have our life's greatest accomplishment in Africa, our climb should benefit Africa. And if it was for Africa, I decided it should help the AIDS crisis there.

I had been moved by Bono's words, "(AIDS) That's not a cause. That's an emergency." Truth be told, I would be moved by anything the U2 front man had to say. If there's one guy who I would veer from my wedding vows for, it would be Bono. There's something so sexy, so amazing about a guy who can sing and save the world.

Bono had my attention, and thank goodness he turned it to something serious. I went to his website, www.data.org, and the numbers of the AIDS crisis were staggering. Every day in Africa, HIV/AIDS kills 6,600 people, 8,800 people are infected with the HIV virus, and 1,400 newborn babies are infected during childbirth or by their mothers' milk.

I wanted to do something. Now I could. I searched on Google: "AIDS, Africa, fundraiser, Kilimanjaro climb."

Global Alliance for Africa's 2007 Kilimanjaro Climb to benefit Children Orphaned by HIV/AIDS popped up as a response.

It seemed like a good match. Global Alliance for Africa is a small, Chicago-based non-profit that partners with African-based organizations, fostering real change in people's lives there. They focused on the needs of vulnerable children, particularly those left behind by the HIV/AIDS-related death of their parents. After all, there were thirteen million of them in Africa, more than the population of New Jersey and Vermont combined.

Signing up for Global Alliance for Africa's climb would be beyond just taking a trip and making a reservation for the next jaunt up the mountain. In addition to paying for our trip, we needed to raise $10,000 for the organization's AIDS orphans programs.

It would be have to be a very public, exposed endeavor.

Raising $10,000, when sometimes I was left with just $5 in my bank account, would mean reaching out to just about everyone Chris and I knew, telling them our mission and asking for their support. It seemed worth it.

Still, it took a couple of months for me to call Global Alliance for Africa, requesting more information about the climb. Sam, a Global Alliance for Africa project coordinator, told me she just returned from the organization's 2006 trip. They made their summit attempt starting at midnight under a full moon. I got goose bumps.

She told me about the organization's mission to provide three meals a day, a safe home environment, education through a secondary school, access to health care and psycho-social support to orphans. I was hooked.

Sam's e-mail was loaded with attachments, including an itinerary detailing the organization's Kilimanjaro climb set to leave in February 2007. The group would take the Rongai Route, the path on the side of the mountain closest to Kenya.

I told Sam that I wanted to go, but I'd get back to her.

Months past as I got swept up in a family issue that required several trips to Vermont. I stopped exercising as much-and spent a lot of energy on phone calls trying to figure out the next steps.

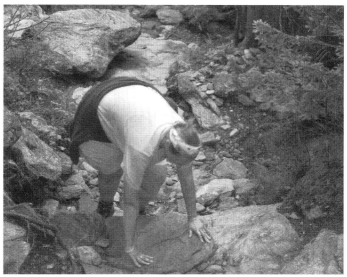

My punishing trek up Mount Mansfield showed I had a lot more training to do before Kilimanjaro.

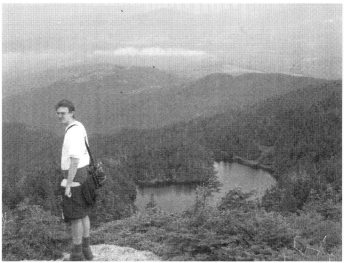

Chris standing above the Lake of the Clouds.

The less I exercised, the worse I slept. The worse I slept, the more I worried. The more I worried, the less I exercised. My weight was creeping up again-first two pounds, then five pounds, then ten pounds.

During one trip to Vermont, my friend Megan and I decided we needed some air. We took my niece and nephew, age five and seven, up Mount Philo, a 650-foot hill. My niece, wearing sandals, stayed with us during the climb. My nephew practically ran to the picnic tables at the summit. We ate double-decker sandwiches and cheese puffs that I carried in my picnic backpack.

As I tucked my niece in bed that night, she crouched forward, pulling the covers over her, "Remember when we were on the mountain?"

"Wasn't it great?" I said, brushed her blond hair out of her eyes and eased her head back onto the pillow. She drifted off to sleep. It was great, and it was time to get back to my mountain climbing mission.

A few weeks later, I asked Chris to come with me to Vermont. It was close enough to my thirty-second birthday that I thought a Camel's Hump hike would be a great way to celebrate. We drove to Vermont, but the torrential rain made it far too dangerous to attempt.

In July, I talked Chris into coming to Vermont with me again, despite the family drama that consumed me. This time, I said, we'd try Vermont's highest peak, Mount Mansfield. There was additional incentive. It was the same weekend as the Vermont Brewer's Festival, an annual summer celebration of microbrew beer on the Lake Champlain waterfront in Burlington.

The Abnaki Indians called Mount Mansfield "Moze-o-de-be-Wadso," for "Mountain with the head of a moose." These days, people say it looks like the profile of a man's face.

We took the Long Trail from Smuggler's Notch to traverse from the Adam's apple to the summit. By the time I had hiked four hours and made it to the chin (4,393'), my thighs were raw and tender. I shuddered and froze as I maneuvered over more exposed, windy parts of the mountain. I imagined missing a step and tumbling my way down the mountain, eventually being pierced by an evergreen.

Chris stayed with me, telling me where he lodged his foot on the rock, before pushing himself upward. When I was especially stuck, he'd extend his hand down and pull me up. We scrambled over boulders, up the side of the mountain, and finally made it to the summit, the top of Mount Mansfield's chin. We walked carefully to avoid the state's largest swath of arctic tundra. We looked out around a sea of mountains, none taller than where we were standing.

I was sore, really sore, but a storm was on the way and we needed to get down the mountain.

About an hour into our descent, we realized we somehow missed a turn and instead of taking the summit ridge down, we were on the Laura Cowles Trail, a nearly vertical chute of wobbly rocks, down the exact opposite side of the mountain from where we started.

The sky was getting dark. After reading about a cairn called Frenchman's Pile, dedicated to a man killed by a lightning bolt near the summit, we decided it was best not to turn back to go up and over the mountain. Really, I was happy with the decision because I didn't want to do any extra hiking. I looped my arm around trees for balance because my leg muscles weren't much help for stability.

As we neared the bottom of the trail, I called my older brother Bryan, who lived nearby, begging him to come pick us up. He did, and we were more than grateful. As soon as we reached the Underhill State Park waiting area, it started to rain. It took Bryan forty-five minutes by car to circle the mountain and return us to where we parked that morning. Imagine if we had to walk!

Our reward for the trek-mountain mishaps and all—was going to the Vermont Brewers Festival—a gathering of great microbreweries along Lake Champlain.

Even the microbrew sampling that night didn't quell my muscles much. While I was glad to have hiked Vermont's highest peak, an accomplishment we toasted over God-knows-how-many-mini-glasses of beer, I knew it was time to get serious about my training if I wanted to climb Kilimanjaro.

When I returned to New Jersey, I winced for a week while walking. I planned my hikes in my calendar, in addition to five days a week at the gym. It was a mix of cardio for endurance, weight training for strength, and yoga for balance and flexibility.

Chris and I started hiking regularly again. By the end of the summer, I felt committed enough in my training to climb Kilimanjaro. I started to relish (not dread) a good workout. My legs felt ready to pounce. I was re-energized and motivated.

I taped a photo of Kilimanjaro on my refrigerator and next to my computer screen to remind me of my goal. I thought about being on top of the mountain every day. In September, I sent in our deposit for the Kilimanjaro trip. It was time to tell people what we were up to.

I built a website, www.fatwomanonthemountain.com, posted "Before" and "After" photos of myself, told my weight loss story and Global Alliance for Africa's purpose. I drafted a letter that would be e-mailed and mailed to everyone we knew asking them to contribute. I was finally putting myself out there.

Since my husband was hosting a party for his running group, the Summit Hash House Harriers (they like to call themselves "drinkers with a running problem"), I figured it would be a good time to start garnering support for our trip.

I printed out a photo of Kilimanjaro and posted it to my refrigerator, marking the middle with fund-raising benchmarks, like a giant thermometer through the middle of the mountain.

They came over, and people asked again and again about the trip.

"How are you going to train?"

"How long will it take you?"

"What if only one of you makes it to the top?" (I figured they meant Chris.)

By the end of the party, I knew I ate too much: three jumbo cookies—one chocolate chunk, one oatmeal raisin, one white chocolate macadamia nut. Then there were two margaritas, three beers, and two bowls of chili (each with a cornbread square).

I think that's it—except a peapod or two while I was setting out the veggie platter, thinking, *I should really avoid the cookies tonight.*

When I cleaned up after the party, it took all the willpower I had to not lick the chili left on the side of the pot, now dotted in soap. Anxiety was getting the best of me and I knew it. The simmering sensation made me want to jump out of my own skin and run far, far away.

Because of my big, fat mouth, most people in my office knew I intended to climb Kilimanjaro. My website drew as many as a thousand visitors in a day.

Simply giving up on that kind of quest—the kind that people latch on to, and live vicariously through you—wouldn't pass unnoticed. I had to do it no matter what my mind said about it.

Everyone was watching. *What if I failed?*

I needed to come up with a plan. I had to actually send out the fundraising letter.

I started making a list of people to ask for donations. My mind did a roll call of everyone I ever knew. I started with friends and family.

I thought about people who haven't seen me in a decade or so, opening the letter and laughing at the thought of me climbing Kilimanjaro. If they could do any math, and if they knew that my top weight was 360, they would think I was far too heavy to take on this challenge. I thought some of my old coworkers would receive and open the letters together, taking time to share stories with new reporters: "Kara was so fat ..."

Or perhaps they would be proud and supportive. I hoped they would be that way, but human nature leads so many to pick apart someone's faults. Fat is such an easy target.

I wondered whether my friend who had gastric bypass surgery would be supportive. She and I have lost about the same amount, except her insurance company will pay for her to get "nipped and tucked." Meanwhile, my thighs looked like an eighty-year-old elephant's after the weight loss.

Enough about family, what about businesses? I thought about the kinds of places I've frequented in the past. There were all of those Vermont bagel shops where I worked, that all-you-can-eat buffet restaurant.

I thought the folks at the pharmacy might recognize me and

contribute, after my many minutes standing in the candy aisle looking for something to self-medicate. I thought about the bread bakery, next to my former newspaper bureau in Brighton, Michigan. Even though I organized our office's healthy lunches, a weekly healthy meal for people trying to lose weight, I stopped in the bakery almost daily because the bakery offered free slices of bread. Most times the bread was warm, straight from the oven, and it went well with a cube of butter in the nearby crock. Then there was the neighboring candy store, where I got my daily stash of Swedish Fish and Swedish Berries. Sometimes, since I had so little money, I paid for a few dollars in candy using loose change.

Could these people, who I chose as my pushers, be my Kilimanjaro supporters?

I scrapped the list of businesses-because I wasn't going back there again-and focused on friends and family. I sent out our first batch of e-mails to family and friends in October.

Some family members, such as my mother-in-law Robin, forwarded the letter to their friends.

> *Dear family and friends,*
>
> *I'm sharing with you the good heart and ambitious goals of our son Christopher and his wife Kara. It's all about helping even a few of the thirteen million (the number takes my breath away!) AIDS orphans in Africa. Please take a few minutes and click on a few links and learn about our crazy kids and the Global Alliance for Africa. Your dollars go directly to the charity. Christopher and Kara are covering their own costs (including ankle bandages and foot balm) from their own piggy bank. If you can help, then the children (ours and Africa's) thank you.*

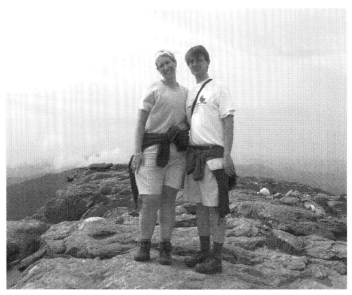

On top of Mount Mansfield, Vermont's highest peak.

We made our pledge deadline December 1, World AIDS Day, figuring the blast of media attention would spur people to action.

Still, in the first few weeks of the fundraising, I was a little nervous as only a handful of donations trickled in online and through the mail.

I planned two fundraising events, hikes though our favorite stomping grounds, including Jockey Hollow and Mount Tammany, a mountain along the Delaware Water Gap, separating New Jersey from Pennsylvania.

A few people said they'd come to the Delaware Water Gap hike, but as the day grew closer, people cancelled. Eventually everyone did, except my *Courier News* coworker Brandon.

Brandon, who was raised on a farm in Lancaster, Pennsylvania, is the kind of coworker you want to have. He's young, ambitious, and able. As a person, he's as good as a home-made blueberry pie at a Pennsylvania country store.

I adored Brandon but since he was the only person committed to the hike, I thought about canceling the event.

It was humiliating that after sending an e-mail out to more than one hundred people in and around New Jersey, only one was willing to support us by hiking with us. Did that mean no one believed in us? Did I believe in us?

I worried I made a huge mistake and would have to somehow come up with thousands of dollars of donations, in addition to the costs of our trip. Should I listen to this lack of support as a sign that I shouldn't be hiking?

In the end, Chris and I decided we needed to hike anyway. So we gave Brandon good directions. He brought his fiancée Abby, their dog Harper, and their friend Lisa. I put a note on my car in case someone else came, but they didn't.

We walked into the forest together and headed up the red dot trail, a short but steep jaunt up the mountain. Harper, a puppy at the time, would run ahead, circle back and to Brandon and Abby's "Here, girl!" calls. This was my first hiking trip with someone other than Chris, so I worried that they would go too fast for me. But they didn't. We walked and talked the whole way up the mountain, an hour-long trek that took us to the summit with sweeping views of the Delaware River (and Interstate 80) below.

The blue trail took us down the mountain, a winding, relaxed path by a rushing waterfall, leading to the river. Harper made her way into the water and shook vigorously, nearly showering us in eau de wet dog.

When we finished, I opened the trunk of my car, which was loaded with granola bars, cheese sticks, and apple cider for our end-of-trail tailgate. They handed me a $100 check made to Global Alliance for Africa, our first big donation.

Brandon, Abby, and Lisa were the only people who came to our second hike at Jockey Hollow. Instead of being a fundraiser, it was just a walk with friends. I wasn't so worried at that point because the donations were trickling in.

A letter campaign, a couple in-person solicitations, and a few more e-mail blasts later (right before the World AIDS Day deadline, of course), we exceeded our goal with pledges and donations of more than $11,000 to Global Alliance for Africa. It felt like a glowing endorsement of what we were about to do.

With the fundraising behind us, Chris and I could focus on training for the final two months.

We collected advice about hiking Kilimanjaro. We e-mailed friends-of-friends who had reached its summit to get an idea of what we were in for, all the things the guide books couldn't tell us.

In previous adventures, I've learned that it's the little things that make a big difference. I'll be forever grateful to my former boss Steve's advice before my descent into the Grand Canyon: "Cut your toenails." (If you don't, they'll bang against your boots, and you'll lose a toenail or ten.) So I thought it would be best to collect all sorts of advice from those who dared to climb Kilimanjaro.

We met with the wife of Chris' former boss, an uber-athlete, who kept up with the porters during her trek the prior summer. She passed along her books *Kilimanjaro: To the Roof of Africa* and *Far from Help!* (a wilderness survival guide). Both books freaked me out.

I reached out to mountain mavens such as a woman who hiked to raise money for a journalism fellowship in her late husband's name. Our Himalayan-hiking friend-of-the-family suggested we contact her friend Allison, who had climbed up and down Kilimanjaro in 4.5 days the prior summer. It was during her honeymoon.

Her advice was plentiful:

~ Get your legs as strong as possible.

~ Take Diamox (to alleviate the effects of the altitude).

~ Never be without ChapStick.

~ Bring lots of high quality socks.

~ Buy toe warmers and hand warmers.

~ Take lots of wipes because you'll be six days without a shower.

~ Take toilet paper, though the toilets will leave much to be desired.

~ Organize your things in ZipLoc bags since you won't think clearly at 18,000 feet.

~ Bring energy bars-they'll be the only thing you can stomach in the altitude.

~ Have hard-sole slippers so you have something to slip your tired feet into other than your stiff boots.

Something that Allison e-mailed stuck with me:

"Let me tell you that you will make it. Kili is not technical, it is just a long hike, and your route has lots of time built in for altitude adjustment. Your mind will get you before your body—just be aware of that—it always does."

I used Allison's advice to train my mind while I was training my body. Every time I was on the stair stepper, every time I meditated in yoga class, I thought of myself climbing the mountain, and eventually reaching the summit. I taped another picture of Kilimanjaro, this one with two elephants grazing in front of it, to my computer at work. I changed my log-on password to Uhuru Peak.

As exciting as it was, around Christmas time when holiday cards accumulated in our mailbox (though we hadn't sent out a single one), I started to dread training, which took at least two hours before I went to work each morning.

In addition to the journey before us, we had to move out of our apartment by New Year's Day so our landlords could convert the two-family home to a one-family of their own.

My friend Jessica was in town for the holidays, and she invited me out for one of our traditional Starbucks outings. At first, I was hesitant: the to-do list was piling up and I could only run 3.5 miles, when most people suggested that I should be able to run at least four miles to prepare for the hike. I begrudged every minute of moving since the Kilimanjaro climb was only seven weeks away.

Though moving was a wonderful training exercise for us, after lugging boxes down from the attic-pushing the weight limits of boxes with my extensive Martha Stewart magazine collection—and eventually loading and unloading a moving truck, I needed a break.

It was four days after Christmas, and I had come off my holiday sugar high back into training. I was frazzled, and Jessica knew it. I talked in spurts about all that was frustrating me. Packing was taking too long. Chris played guitar while I packed plates.

I descended into self-doubt. I talked about how some proprietors of success say that a woman must put herself on the line to be really great. Here I was in a mind-bendingly vulnerable position.

In Starbucks, I had a fat-free, decaf, sugar-free vanilla latte—reminding me of everything I couldn't have. Jessica had tea, a venti-size cup of Calm. Jessica was my friend who passed the Connecticut bar while working full-time. She was my ambassador of calm. We met during a Weight Watchers meeting four years before. Her weight was hovering above 200 pounds. Mine was stuck at about 305. We sympathized with each other's weight loss woes in the parking lot and agreed to exchange e-mail addresses, reminding each other to be good during the week.

The next week, we went to a Weight Watchers meeting and then to Starbucks. In some of our earlier Starbucks outings we used to have low-fat muffins. Then we found out how many calories they contained. Then we kept to low-fat lattes and conversation.

Jessica and I were about one hundred pounds apart in our weight loss struggle, but we had mutual understanding of each other's obsessions. Sometimes she'd talk about how she couldn't stop until she got to the end of a bag—and I thought she might have seen me in the pantry the day before.

We both came from broken homes. We both ate to deal with that and just about every other life uncertainty or complication.

We kept in touch via e-mail when I moved to Michigan so Chris could earn his MBA. Then she went to Connecticut to go to law school, and eventually practice. Each time she's back in New Jersey, we try to get together for a workout or Starbucks date. I wished Jessica lived closer. She makes me think I'm not so crazy.

About a week after my Starbucks outing with Jessica, Chris and I had moved out of our apartment, and I found an orange mailing envelope from Jessica marked "Kili Care Package" on my new doorstep.

I pulled out the note:

> *Kara,*
>
> *It was so good to see you the other day–you always have the ability to bring focus and clarity to my crazy hectic life. I think it's so utterly amazing that you are making this trek to the tippy top of Africa. It's going to be an unbelievable journey! I have absolutely no doubt it'll be a goal you'll blow away.*
>
> *So in honor of you and hopefully to bring some focus and clarity to your life, I've put together a Kili Care Package–a package of goodies designed to help make the next few weeks of preparation all that more interesting and easy.*

I pulled out the package of about a dozen Calm tea bags, packaged together in a ZipLoc bag.

Jessica also sent a workout log and two CD mixes—one for working out and one for hanging out.

> *So you've got just a handful of weeks left but I'm cer-tain you'll be at the top of that mountain!*
>
> *I hope all these goodies help–say hi to the god of Mount Kilimanjaro for me!*
>
> *Love, Jessica*

I boiled some water and had a cup of Calm.

6. GEARING UP

Many retailers seem to think it is fine for a 3XL man to have an outdoor adventure. However, it seemed they couldn't imagine a woman of my girth going out in the wild.

Global Alliance for Africa sent a two-page checklist of gear to buy. Since a Kilimanjaro is like a trek from the Equator to the North Pole, we'd need a little bit of everything. It meant digging through our camping gear, and learning that I would have to buy just about everything.

Five weeks before the trip, I was still without a sturdy, hooded jacket and snow pants—items I dreaded buying because of my unusual size.

My upper half responded well to weight loss—so much so, that I could buy shirts at The Gap and other normal-sized shops. My lower body dropped as well—from a size 32 to a 22 or 24. It is a sizable drop but not enough to fit into a women's XL, the biggest size carried in most sporting goods stores.

We hit Bill's Army Navy, a sporting goods store in Millburn, so Chris could look for sturdier boots. Meanwhile, I hit the snow pants rack.

I let out a "Yes!" outburst as I found a pair of XXL men's snow pants and held them. They were a good six inches longer than I needed them to be, but I tried to pull them over my jeans, thinking that I would need them to fit over layers.

I pulled the full length between my ankle and my calf, and then I inched upward. My thighs filled every cubic inch they offered. Then I got to my great barrier hips with little alternating tugs, one in the back, one in the front, and over again. The pants fit over my hips-that is, with the zipper undone and the pockets popped open.

Men's clothing is too narrow to accommodate a woman's hips or thighs. Well, at least my hips.

I caught myself thinking that I could lose another ten pounds or enough inches around my hips in time for these to pull on smoothly. Reality check: weight loss doesn't work that way. These pants wouldn't fit. I need to be limber, strong, and steady—not worried that my pants would burst open in the face of a climber behind me—that is, if any would be slower than me.

I pushed the pants down in a defeated heap on the floor before any sales people could come back to ask how they fit. I clipped the pants back on the hanger, a troublesome task since the thick Gore-Tex fabric had to be doubled because the pants were so big. I returned to Chris, where the sales person had him trying on too-short, too-wobbly boots for the adventure in front of us.

Our next stop was Blue Ridge Mountain Sports in Madison, an upscale commuter town, where just about every customer who came in that Saturday asked for a North Face jacket of some kind. I was no different. The North Face was a close second to the healthy status symbol of the Nalgene-bottle look at college. I always wanted to have one.

Growing up in Vermont, my grandmother always bought

my winter coats. I remember thumbing through the racks, looking for coats that the well-off kids had. Sometimes I'd try to squeeze into overcoats in regular-kids sizes, trying to convince my grandmother that the outerwear could go unbuttoned until I lost weight.

Back then, as generous as my grandmother was to me, The North Face was out of our price range. When I was old enough to buy my own jackets, they were out of my size range.

Now, I was skinnier and I was going to finally have The North Face jacket of my dreams. The Kilimanjaro jacket requirements were: "Shell jacket with hood-breathable Gore-Tex or similar product. Must be large enough to fit over layers."

My worry was whether an expedition-style jacket would be big enough to fit over my hips. I started with a large jacket. Then, an extra-large.

Finally, an extra-extra-large jacket fit. I imagined The North Face jackets are typically slender on its uber-fit customers. So, I took this in stride.

I caught myself thinking that I just needed it as a top layer—perhaps it could be left open. I stopped myself before my thoughts got any sillier. If I were to hike Kilimanjaro, winds bustling at minus 25 degrees, I would need to be able to zip my coat. I was buying a Summit Series jacket—at $298, the jacket is designed to withstand a mountain's worst elements. It doesn't promise to function if it's left open.

I swam in the top part of my jacket. Its sleeves hung far below my hands. The hips were snug. But I was in a North Face and it felt great.

More than anything, I needed to look the part of the hiker. I still had some convincing to do for myself to understand that I was ready for this. It didn't help that I was asked, "Have you

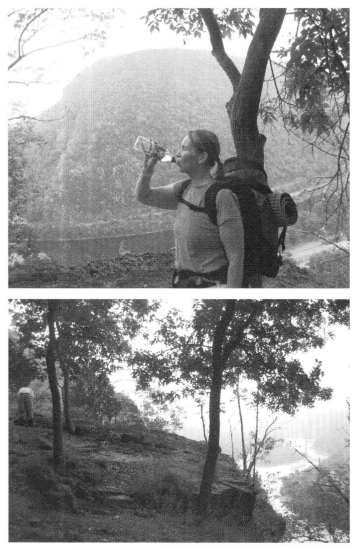

Drinking up and enjoying the view of the Delaware River (and Interstate 80!) from Mount Tammany in the Delaware Water Gap National Park.

done any serious hiking before?" in just about every sporting goods store.

I found myself announcing details about our past adventures immediately, cutting salespeople's assumption off at the pass before I started asking for products. This was typically a recap of the previous year's jaunt down and back up the Grand Canyon, followed by Zion and Bryce in subsequent days. Sometimes people looked at me with disbelief. It was like I could see them

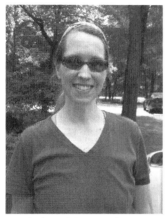

Ready for a hike in Jockey Hollow National Park.

thinking, I bet she did climb the canyon-on a mule's back.

As Chris tested out a pair of boots by walking laps around the wool sweaters and long johns, I gravitated, as I typically do, toward "one-size-really-fits-all" items in outfitter stores. I felt less antsy looking at sunglasses, fleece sleeping caps, and socks.

Since I am a chronic sunglasses loser, I settled on a $40 red-rimmed Optic Nerve pair. So, there it was; everything that

I would wear on top would be from the serious gear stores. The bottom half would have to be from plus-sized stores.

For snow pants, I clicked through Junonia's website, which was for plus-sized adventurers like myself. Anne Kelly founded Junonia in 1995. At size 16, Kelly was sick of having to wear clunky, heavy sweat suits in her step aerobics classes, while her thin classmates had more comfortable, movable attire. Kelly had a hard time getting investors for her active-wear catalog for plus-size women. People balked at the idea, saying, "If they were active, they would be small. So where's the market?"

A dozen years later, Kelly's company boasts millions in sales, split between active and casual wear offerings. She hears from customers who are marathon runners, tri-athletes, English Channel swimmers, dogsled racers, dragon boat crewmembers and search and rescue workers. Her company carries everything from plus-size swimwear (her number one seller), bicycle shorts, tennis getups and yes, snow pants.

When my pair of snowpants arrived, it seemed they were built for my butt. That's because they were.

It was time to outfit my insides for Africa—so we visited the travel doctor.

I worried the appointment with a travel doctor would begin with him balking at our request to talk about altitude medications to climb Kilimanjaro, since I was still a bit of a giant. I worried he would ask me to step on the scale before meeting us.

I don't know why I fear doctors so much, but the more people I meet who have weight issues, the more I notice this. We tend to fear those who are working to keep us healthy, as if we just don't want to hear the guilt trip. I worry a doctor won't understand the internal struggle that plagues me, making my weight loss battle far more complicated than just eating less and moving more.

But this doctor wasn't that sort at all. He was lean, but seemed to be a softy. His suit was an unassuming gray, a summer-weight fabric on a winter's day. I wondered if he was a retired physician, passing the time between Doctors Without Borders stints in this otherwise bland medical complex.

With ice-blue eyes, he looked over the report he prepared,

to tell us what ailments we could expect to encounter in Tanzania.

"You must hear about some pretty exotic adventures," Chris said to him, as he scanned the document detailing how many shots and prescriptions we'd need.

"Kilimanjaro is about as exotic as it gets—at least, as far as immunizations go," he said, casting a slight smile, knowing we, not he, were the ones about to get poked.

The first on the list was yellow fever, a deadly disease spread by the mosquito. Its symptoms include a fever, jaundice, the shutdown of your kidney, liver, or lungs, and vomiting blood.

"And we're just getting started," the doctor said, seeming to take pleasure in the number of shots and pills prescribed from his office.

Fortunately, Chris and I had a full battery of immunizations before an international trip two years previously. My arm felt like a colander after the yellow fever, hepatitis A and tetanus shots. We also had to take an oral typhoid vaccination, which felt like swallowing a dark dose of evil, sitting swirling in your stomach. A rabies vaccination was also on his list—though he said we would be fine without it.

"If you get bit by one of the cats over there, rabies will be the least of your worries," he smiled.

I gulped.

He wasn't done. He still had to send us with parting gifts— prescriptions.

In Tanzania, the risk for malaria, a mosquito-borne illness, is everywhere. The parasite in the bloodstream makes you feel like you have the flu. Left untreated, you may develop jaundice and eventually fall into a coma. Even at the best medical facilities, ten percent of people with malaria die. We wouldn't be allowed to travel with Global Alliance for Africa if we didn't have a malaria pill.

Malarone was his suggestion; it doesn't have the delirium associated with Larium. And since we would be 200 miles south of the equator, doxycycline, which can make people sensitive to the sun, wouldn't work either.

The doctor took out the blue pad and a series of stamps from a desk drawer.

"This is my favorite part of my day," he said, lining them up in front of him.

With malaria addressed, he said it was time to talk about the ailment we'd encounter in Africa: traveler's diarrhea. For that, he gave a preventative prescription for Cipro, which we would take if we found ourselves hitting the toilets four or five times a day.

Then came the issue of altitude. Diamox is the standard among climbing crowds. The trouble was it typically doesn't sit well with those who are allergic to sulfa drugs. I am allergic to sulfa drugs. Fortunately, there was an alternative, dexamethasone. "Dex"—as it's called in climbing crowds—is a steroid. When the doctor first mentioned Dex, my mind went immediately to the slightly ridiculous movie Vertical Limit, which I secretly love because Chris O'Donnell is in it. There, stranded climbers try to decide who gets the few remaining doses of Dex.

In my case, the steroid would be in far smaller doses than in the emergency kits of climbing guides. I would need to start with a 4 mg pill, allowing the steroid to level out as I got to the summit and stop once I was at a breathing-friendly altitude.

The doctor finished filling out my last prescription and ripped it off the pad. We took the stack of scripts and headed to the pharmacy.

7. ALTITUDE AND ATTITUDE TRAINING

When I announced my intentions to climb Kilimanjaro in the form of a fundraising e-mail, my high school friend Heather responded with the subject: "Wow."

Heather was never afraid to be Heather. She was an art student, and creativity flowed through her being. Heather, with her bright blue eyes and freckled ever-sunblocked skin, was a snowboarding instructor in Telluride, Colorado. If she were a rock star, she would be Bjork, and never spared energy worrying about what other people thought of her. I admired, maybe even envied, her ability to live in the mountains, free from corporate life.

Heather is incredibly intelligent and creative. She graduated top of her class in graphic design at Syracuse University and her career catapulted into a top firm in Boston. A few years into her career, we met for a mini-vacation in Winter Park, Colorado, where a few of my college pals worked after they graduated. They loved life on the even bigger mountains than the ones in Vermont and competed for the most runs in a ski season.

About a year after our Winter Park venture—where I tore the meniscus in my knee during a beginner skiing lesson—Heather decided she wanted more Colorado skiing. The next year, she signed up for Telluride's (now defunct) Triple Threat Snowboarding clinic as a twenty-fifth birthday gift to herself. After the week's worth of lessons, she was hooked and asked her instructor if she had the makings to teach.

He responded, "Hell, yes. Get your ass out here." Shortly thereafter, she submitted her resignation from her graphic design job to be on the slopes full time.

Eight seasons later, when it came time for my Kilimanjaro climb, Heather had all sorts of outdoor certifications. She was avalanche trained and wilderness-rescue ready.

When Heather learned of my Kilimanjaro quest, we exchanged mountain adventure stories. I went through my standard list of prequalifications like I did with most people who had only seen me when I was really, really fat. I could tell she was concerned that I was over my head when it came to Kilimanjaro.

She asked, "How is it that you go from hiking a few mountains in Vermont, the Grand Canyon, and then Kilimanjaro?"

Heather had climbed Mount Rainier, a shorter but far more technically demanding feat in Washington State. She was spending her summers as a wilderness guide and seemed to be more of an expert on the subject than me. Our online correspondence shifted to altitude, which was my biggest Kilimanjaro fear. If it weren't for the altitude, climbing Kilimanjaro would be a very, very long walk. That long walk takes you to where the air is half as thin as it is at sea level. The thinner the air, the lower the oxygen level in your blood. Your body doesn't like being oxygen-deprived. Your body tries to overcompensate with the condition known as hypoxia.

In high altitude, the brain may swell with blood. The lungs could swim in fluid, making it impossible to inhale the super thin air. You could become sick. You could even die.

People can feel sick with mild altitude sickness symptoms such as a headache or a smidge of nausea as low at about 5,000. It is almost unavoidable above 11,500 feet.

My friend Jessica told me she wanted to curl up on the trail and take a nap while hiking a 14,000-foot mountain in Colorado. I was headed to Kilimanjaro's 19,343-foot summit, where a hiker can typically manage a half-step or two before becoming winded.

My highest climbs were in Vermont. They were beautiful but made me feel like a flatlander compared to the terrain I would be traversing. I lived at sea level. The mighty Camel's Hump stands at 4,083 feet. The highest point in Vermont was Mount Mansfield at 4,393 feet. While I was fine during my stays in Winter Park years before, I had made it to the top of ski trails via a chairlift. I was just coasting down them in a "pizza" wedge wider than the kiddy lessons around me.

Heather's home in Mountain Village, a neighboring town of Telluride, was at about 9,500 feet. Her highest climb was Rainier, at 14,410 feet. I trusted her expertise about thin air. She lived and breathed it.

Even on her Rainier trip, several young hikers had to turn back, or worse, got pegged in sleeping bags to the ice-slicked mountainside and were told to wait until the rest of the group returned for them.

I had an idea of booking a trip to Denver shortly before the climb and then running on a treadmill for a weekend. So I wrote to Heather, asking what she thought.

I could almost hear her laughing at me in her e-mail response:

FAT WOMAN ON THE MOUNTAIN

A better plan (although probably not as do-able) is to come spend three weeks in Denver (5,800')/Telluride or Mountain Village (8,750' or 9,450')/Leadville (your best bet and possibly the cheapest option)/Rocky Mountains in general right before you leave. I don't think coming up to Denver a month beforehand to run on a treadmill will do much for you, except maybe bruise your ego if you don't acclimatize well.

Heather explained that it takes her about three days to become seventy-five percent acclimatized to high altitude areas. The idea of altitude training in Telluride stuck with me. I knew I needed to take myself seriously when it came to this journey.

Her harrowing high-altitude stories made me decide to spend a week hiking up Telluride's snow-covered slopes to get a feel of what it was to work with less oxygen. In Telluride, the air pressure is about two-thirds what it is at sea level. On Kilimanjaro, it would be about half. The town itself was at about 10,000 feet. The tallest peaks I could climb there during in the winter were about 12,000 feet.

Our Kilimanjaro climb would begin at 6,397 feet, slightly higher than the mile-high city of Denver. Our first day of climbing would end at Moorland Camp, which sits at 8,530 feet. After four more days of going up, we would summit at 19,340 feet.

Heather, who has a tiny studio apartment stocked with ski equipment, set me up with her friends Joanna and Dennis. Joanna and Dennis, who teach skiing at Telluride in the winter and lead wilderness trips in Durango during the summer, became my altitude instructors of sorts.

When I looked online, I found a $292 direct plane ticket

from Newark to Telluride/Montrose airport. It felt like a sign.

I spent the next few weeks charting out days on a calendar—trying to figure out which days I could spare-paid or unpaid—in the days before the trip to Africa.

Chris thought the idea was completely unnecessary. But I pushed on with my plans, even though I worried he would resent me once we climbed to 12,000 feet on Kilimanjaro, the highest I could safely hike in the Telluride area in winter conditions.

Why not have a little altitude advantage? Chris always out-performed me. Most times, even after the bulk of my weight loss, I felt I might be holding him back as he slowed on hikes, waiting for me around the bend. I wanted to keep up this time, even if it was at a half-step pace.

I wrote back to Heather, asking if ten days would be enough.

"Some altitude training is better than none," she replied.

I pulled together every possible personal and vacation day and handed two consecutive vacation requests-one for Telluride, one for Africa-to my editor, who rolled his eyes but then signed off on them anyway. My Telluride trip would be January 27 to February 6. That would give me ten days in thin air. I would return two days before I'd leave for Africa, February 9. Our climb started on February 13.

The trip to Telluride would have to be on a tight budget. I had sunk my resources into my gear, and I still had at least $200 more to spend. About $50 of that would be Smart Wool socks alone—but it was worth it to have top-of-the-line socks for the tough journey ahead.

I clipped coupons for soup, egg whites, veggie burgers, salad, and other supplies that I thought I would need in town. I packed enough oatmeal for each morning and a box of whole wheat pasta, thinking that could save a couple of bucks at the mountain top resort area where the rich and famous—Tom Cruise, Oprah, and Ralph Lauren—have been known to frolic. Mountainside villas were selling in the $10 million range. From most pictures, the town of Telluride looks like a movie set with posh restaurants and spas. I wouldn't be visiting either during my trip.

~~~

Packing my suitcase was practice for packing for Africa. I brought long underwear, fleece jackets, a down liner, my jacket, and hiking poles. I wore my hiking boots on the plane because that was the one piece of luggage I couldn't afford to lose.

Unlike most of the passengers on my direct flight from Newark to Montrose, Colorado, I didn't bring skis. I loved skiing but my injury rate on the slopes is about 1:3. There have been torn meniscus in my knee, a hurt hand (which I swore was broken until after a member of the ski patrol personally towed my 317-pound body in a sled down the mountain), and other various sore spots. With three weeks until the Kilimanjaro climb, I couldn't afford an injury.

My ten days would be spent hiking in Telluride and Mountain Village, two towns that sit within the San Juan range—a relatively young set of mountains with jagged peaks that haven't had a chance to be worn with time.

For that reason, the San Juan mountains have tight clusters of 14,000-foot peaks. Since I didn't have the equipment or the skills to do winter mountaineering, I decided to limit my hiking to the ski slopes, which went as high as 12,255 feet-still more than 6,000 feet short of Kili's summit.

My first stop after plunking my bags in Joanna and Dennis' home was the market. I felt woozy already, since the prices felt twice as high as sea level! I had brought coupons for my sundries—oatmeal, bread, peanut butter, bananas, and yogurt.

The altitude first affected me in the form of a mild headache and then feeling slightly disorientated at the market. Or, perhaps it was just trying to sort through all those coupons.

My mother called me to make sure my flight went well. I found it tough to talk and shop at the same time. I was confused and the labels on the shelves blurred around me. My twinge of a headache started twisting in my skull. Instead of using the store's bags, I packed my groceries into the same daypack I would be using on Kilimanjaro, figuring that would be weight resistance training. The $90 for a week's supply of food went all the way to the top of the sack. I felt a little teetery, with soup cans pressing against my back.

I thought, I'm in trouble. But then I realized acclimatization was part of the process. It was why I was there. But I was only at about 10,000 feet. Two weeks from then, I would be on my way to Kilimanjaro's 19,343-foot summit.

I took an Advil and took it easy. I retired to the daybed in the Joanna and Dennis' guest room. I pulled out a trail map that I snagged from the information booth. I stared at the green, blue, and black diamond trails as I drifted off to sleep.

I met up with Heather on the morning after I arrived. She made me a brunch of breakfast quesadillas and we talked more about mountains—and about how we now were more self-confident since we had grown up together in South Burlington. After all, in high school I was a benchwarmer on the freshman basketball team, even when I was a sophomore. Heather refused to run in gym class, taking about twenty minutes to walk what should have been a twelve-minute mile.

But now I was about to climb Kilimanjaro. She had just finished a hike and ski adventure in Silverton, Colorado, which had been featured in the New York Times travel section. You could see her hot pink jacket and gray snow pants hiking up the mountain to the most treacherous terrain she had ever skied.

"I keep surprising myself," she said, retreating to the desk of her studio apartment. She returned, smiling gloriously with two ice axes. She had been ice climbing five times at Ice Park, a man-made ice climbing area not far from Telluride. She wanted to eventually climb Bear Creek Falls, a sheath of ice that hung from jagged rocks on the Telluride Ski Resort's backside.

We decided to hike there that afternoon. That way, she could do some reconnaissance work on the area and I could start my hiking schedule with an easy five-mile hike with about a thousand feet of altitude gain.

Heather had a cold that settled in her lungs. Fortunately for me, when it came to lung capacity that meant we were working at about the same pace. Heather stopped to admire an aspen and name the flora round us. She talked about them as if she were introducing friends.

I felt stronger in this second day in Telluride. I was keeping up with Heather, who after we started remembered to tell me, "By the way, we'll be crossing an avalanche field. I've been afraid to take this trail since my Avalanche Level 1 course."

Uh, great.

I felt better as she explained that the chances of a several-ton tumble of snow crushing us was slim, especially because that particular avalanche chute had fallen about a month before.

"And it fell big," she said. We did a little risk assessment, and concluded walking past this avalanche shoot was far safer than driving a car.

"I'd rather die doing something like this than in a car," I said, with faux bravery. In my head I imagined a cold, lonely death under a smothering blanket of snow.

We kept on. I asked all sorts of questions about avalanches on the way there. How do you survive an avalanche?

Her answer: "Pray that someone finds you."

Heather explained there is a ten-minute window between when an avalanche smothers you and when brain damage begins. Your breath melts an ice mask around your mouth, eventually stealing all of the air from you, she explained.

"Oh, ok," I said.

The trail opened with views of the ridges above. We were surrounded by natural winter bliss.

Soon, the avalanche chute was upon us. Heather paused before passing it, saying, "We're safe here."

I looked up at the chute, an open-wide section of mountain where the trees have been knocked over from the force of the snow. A woman died there last year. Heather pointed out where they found her body.

She started up again, this time trudging much faster. I was frustrated that my leg speed was slowed by the altitude, and didn't seem to pick up to match my anxiety. I kept looking up, as if having a couple extra moments to see a wall of white hurling toward me would have saved me. It took a minute to get across the chute, but when it was over, it was like the field never existed.

Surviving our little pass with the avalanche chute gave me a thrill. I was indeed living a little bit more dangerously than before.

I watched people skiing and snowboarding down the other

avalanche chutes on the mountains on the opposite side of the valley. They paused behind a gigantic rock, waiting for other members of the group to catch up, before heading down what looked like a perpendicular sheet of rock and snow.

In the group that came down was one of Heather's mountain co-workers, John. He awaited the rest of his party, reveling in the ride. As they continued down the path we had traversed, I heard a "whoop" coming from them as they passed the avalanche field. Heather congratulated the guys on a good run.

We walked on to Bear Creek Falls, no more than a half-mile up the crunched snow path. Heather put her hand to her forehead to shade her view.

Bear Creek Falls was a gigantic sheath of ice, hanging on the backside of the Telluride Ski Resort. The layer upon layer of ice gave it a blue, sometimes green, shade.

Heather sized up the situation.

"I'd have to hike above the Falls, rappel down them, and climb back up again," Heather said, as she tried to figure how to conquer an area of the falls that is not usually climbed.

She looked excited, not nervous, like me. We each had a Clif Bar and hiked back down the trail, where we barely noticed the avalanche slope this time.

On the way back we ran into a woman hiking solo along the trail, "Tell me it's not much further."

"You're almost there," I said.

"I told myself, 'I am not turning back'," the woman said, as she walked on.

Neither am I, I thought.

~~~

I set my alarm for 6:30 a.m. for my first official day of high altitude training. My right hand dangled outside the three layers of blankets, and the crisp air in my bedroom told me it would be tough to unpeel the covers and get out of bed.

But I wanted to hit the slopes long before the skiers did. That way I could get my uphill panting done out of sight of people coasting down the mountain. Of course, I also figured it would be a lot safer to walk uphill without downhill traffic. I splashed water on my face, dried it off, then slathered 30-SPF sunscreen on my face.

As I was preparing for my first climb up the ski slopes in the kitchen of Dennis and Joanna's home, I pulled out the strawberry jam that I had bought at the market to make a PB&J.

"I should have told you not to buy jam. We have about thirty jars left," Dennis said, walking around the corner.

Dennis and Joanna have a gigantic garden in Durango, where they spend their summers. Dennis makes more than 100 jars of jam for holiday gifts. The jars, with thumbnail-sized hand-written labels, reminded me of my mother's cupboards. Her preserves would last us through the long winters of Canada.

The couple gardened as a way of living; plus, it kept the food bills down in such a tourist destination. A jar of jelly at the market cost $7.

Dennis directed me to the apricot jam that was in the refrigerator, and then pulled a jar of rhubarb plum from the cupboard in case I needed backup. He set out a jar of choke cherry on the counter ledge to send home with me.

I noticed Dennis had been chopping all sorts of dried fruits and nuts on a wooden cutting board, grooved from years of healthy use. He turned to stir the oatmeal cooking on the stove.

It was Dennis's job to make breakfast each morning while Joanna walked the dog Zoe, which is Greek for "life".

As I shook two instant oatmeal packets and emptied them into the bowl, the powder drifted on the tile counter. In the two minutes and forty-five seconds while my breakfast cooked, I wandered to the window, partially caked in frost, where I saw the street lights set a twinkling glitter on the fresh coat of snow. I checked out the digital thermometer, which registered 10 degrees Fahrenheit.

The breakfast routine for Joanna and Dennis was one of togetherness as they reviewed their separate schedules of lessons. I had come on a busy week. Joanna was running a woman's camp, a program celebrating its twenty-fifth year. They often had short-term guests, either hosting friends or making a little extra money renting out the spare room to a short-term ski instructor or drifters like me. But unlike their other guests, instead of asking advice about what trails I was going to ski down, I was asking which ones they thought I should walk up.

When it came to ski trails, Telluride folks seem to be like New Jersey people are when giving directions. Describing ski trails is an art form, especially to Dennis and Joanna, who ditched their day jobs to travel for fourteen months before settling down as ski instructors. That was fourteen years before.

"Skiing is counterintuitive," Dennis said. "People instinctively want to hold back, instead of going with it, falling into the motion. That's why so many beginners fall. They're afraid to let go."

Joanna and Dennis met on 50-mile bike ride. Their second date was a backpacking trip. Dennis had been an engineer, while Joanna was an executive director of a non-profit human service agency. Both were dissatisfied with their career path, and they decided to make a break for it. After more than a year of traveling with the rule of no driving farther than one tank of gas would take them, they decided to start work again, in jobs that felt a lot like play. They bought a mountainside condo seven years ago. Its value had since tripled.

Dennis, who turned fifty-one while I was there, reminded me again and again it was all about the lifestyle. And they were living. He traced his finger along a Telluride ski trail map, helping me match each day of the Kilimanjaro journey with an equivalent training hike in the mountain-high Colorado village. He picked up my well-worn Kilimanjaro itinerary, where I had converted meters to feet, to point out the best Telluride training trails. I had broken them down by day.

His eyes bulged and he looked down, as if to gulp. "Which summit are you going to do?"

"All the way to the top. Uhuru Peak."

"That's going to take …" Dennis said, stopping to find the right words.

I finished for him, "It's going to take everything I've got."

"It's good that you're here. Remember, it's about the journey," Dennis said. He repeated that a number of times. I was sure it was because he thought I wouldn't make it.

I had a plan: Work hard all week to build my high-altitude endurance. I already seemed to do well at about 10,000 feet. It was time to go higher. Since I was there through the Super Bowl, I decided to end a long weekend with Super Hike Sunday, when I would attempt a hike from the bottom of Mountain Village to the very top of See Forever, the highest trail on the mountain at 12,000 feet.

Dennis and I decided a good first solo mission would be Galloping Goose, for however long I could walk it. Galloping

Goose is a green trail, meaning the easiest kind, but it's also Telluride ski resort's longest trail, 4.6 miles to its 11,815-foot top. I set out at 7:30 a.m. While the folks who live around the ski slopes think it's a flat trail, it climbs 2,500 feet. Depending on how well things went, I would be going up to 11,815 feet.

So I set out, as Joanna and Dennis left to take the chondala (half gondola/half chairlift) to the ski school. It was supposed to be a dry day, so I opted to wear my fleece pants, protected to calf-high by gaiters that I swore took fifteen minutes to hitch to my boots. I extended my poles and set off. In the quiet of morning, I made my way up the mountain.

Galloping Goose is a wide, rolling beginner trail-the kind I used to love to ski down. With the slopes not even open yet, I had the trail all to myself, aside from a grooming machine or two that would pass.

I walked, marring the freshly pressed snow, leaving deep footprints on the sides of the trail, mirrored by pole pricks on either side. In most places, the snow was hard and solid under my feet. Other places, my feet sunk, making it seem like I was walking uphill in sand. My thighs would remind me about that later.

Even in the solid spots, I was working harder than I ever had, but moving slower than I ever remembered hiking. My breath sounded like I might be out of shape—like perhaps I was running—but I wasn't. I was just walking slowly up the mountain. I hoped I wasn't getting myself into trouble. Well, if I was, I was at a ski resort, and help would be easy to come by.

I thought for a moment about how or if help would be available on Kilimanjaro. I couldn't imagine it would be. I decided it was best not to panic, not here on the mountain. I reminded myself that I was well trained and ready to take

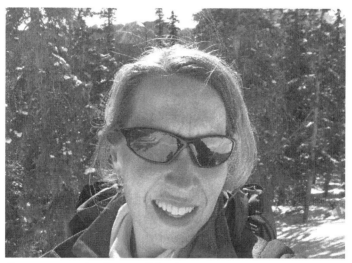

On my way up the slopes in Telluride.

on this path. I had turned up Marmot, a shortcut between one section of Galloping Goose and another. But Marmot was an intermediate trail, and had significantly steeper sections to traverse.

At times my feet slid back, like a running man dance. I plugged my poles into the mountain and lunged forward. One step. Two steps. Move forward.

Once I passed the 10,500 mark, my feet moved significantly slower. I'd find a tree about fifty paces ahead on the trail and tell myself that I could have a break once I reached it. The trail was long and slogging with the crunch of snow underfoot.

I didn't have anyone else with me, so I could break whenever I wanted to. I did a lot, figuring just by being there, by breathing, I was getting stronger. The longer I stayed on the mountain, the better.

I used the "eat-something-every-hour" rule of the Grand Canyon. No, not a full meal, just something—a handful of trail mix, half a Luna bar—something small, about 100 calories, and lots of water. No one told me I should. I just figured it would work. And quite honestly, it gave me an excuse to stop.

But by now, at 9 a.m., the ski lifts had opened and people were coming down the mountain. Some skied out of their mountainside homes, only to ride the chairlift back up again and rush back down again.

It was embarrassing, not being able to move my fastest. Most times, as another skier came down, I'd lose track of my own feet and stumble a bit. The hiking poles got in the way of my own feet. I figured the thin air was making me clumsy.

But seeing the trails in reverse, I was able to enjoy the views of the mountain in winter. I was normally a winter hiking wimp. I could see, and stop to admire Wilson's Peak, a more than 14,000-foot perfectly formed triangle peak, just like it is on the Coors can.

I pressed up the mountain and stopped to rest at the warming huts. Many looked puzzled that I was coming in without doing the ski boot strut-the stiff ankle waddle that it takes to get from one end of a room to another in ski boots.

One skier clunked around in ski boots and said, "I saw you earlier this morning. Did you just walk up here?"

After three very successful hiking days, I decided to make my way from Mountain Village to Telluride, not by gondola, but by foot. I got off to a late start, tired from all the early morning "beat-the-skiers-to-the-mountain" hikes.

There was a trail that cut through the ridge of Mountain Village, sliced through the trees, and ended just south of town. Dennis and Joanna gave me directions. They take that path all the time if they're in the mood to walk to town, a jaunt that takes about an hour going down.

I trudged around town with my red hiking sticks. I looked and felt like the other outdoor adventurers. Indeed, I was. Instead of taking the gondola from Mountain Village to Telluride, I hiked an hour over the ridge to get there.

I spent the afternoon in the library, catching up on writing and reading. I peeled off my layers and connected to the Internet in the cozy Telluride room.

Returning was more difficult, as by 6 p.m. there was no light and a snow squall had started. I decided it was an excellent opportunity to try my miner-like headlamp, a Christmas gift from my mother. I loved that she gave it to me; it was a sign of support for a journey I know worried her.

The headlamp illuminated the snow, making it look like tiny white comets falling everywhere around me. When I hike alone, I hike slowly. Very slowly. My attitude changes with each step. It goes from, "You're balanced and strong," to "When is this hill ever going to end?"

Toward the top I got confused and found myself knee deep in a snow bed. I continued through, ending at the million-dollar condominiums, where I saw some footprints leading to what looked like the right direction. It wasn't quite. I stumbled my way to the neighboring condominium development and then, after realizing my mistake, gingerly slid on the ice-coated driveway, and finally back up the one for Dennis and Joanna's place.

When I arrived, my boots, my snow pants—everything—was caked in snow.

"We were starting to worry about you," Joanna said, as she, Dennis, and Zoe the dog cuddled together for a movie.

Me too, I thought, peeling off my layers, hoping they'd dry by the next day.

~~~

I planned to take the gondola from Mountain Village, up to Station St. Sophia, a crest in the ridge where the free gondola lets skiers out or continues down the other side of the mountain into the town of Telluride. I got out at the top, and set out to conquer See Forever, or at least the steepest, hardest part.

As I stood at its base, it looked like a steep slide, the kind of hill on the Olympics, with professionals barreling down at breakneck speeds, knees bent and bobbling with every movement, arms tucked into their sides.

The hill was pristine after yet another beautiful new snow, so I set out to start walking, up and up. The reward was Giuseppe's Restaurant for lunch, elevation 11,890 feet, where Heather strongly recommended the black bean sauté. She said if I ordered a half-order it would be plenty, and within my budget. I packed some snacks and was looking forward to the break from the PB&Js, no matter how great Dennis's jam was.

I set out, as the ski patrol and mountain staff assembled by the chair lift, and made my way up the long steep hill. My steps were slow. Very slow. I hoped Kilimanjaro wouldn't be this steep because this was really hard. I had a bad feeling it might be.

But stopping wasn't so bad. I'd turn around, exhale deeply, and take in the mountains unfolding all around me. This trail, See Forever, was true to its name.

I felt so blessed to be able to be there, but also to be strong enough to walk there. I gave thanks to my feet, my legs, my heart, and my mind for getting me there and carrying me through this journey. I was so grateful that I was able to make it this far. But two hours up the mountain would be as far as I would get. A ski patrol guy came whooshing down the hill and came to an on-a-dime stop in my path.

"You can't walk up these trails. It's too dangerous," he said. I could tell he was a rule stickler. This was a case of safety first.

I tried to explain my quest, to altitude train so that I'd be ready for Kilimanjaro. My story seemed to interest him as it did most people I encountered, but I still had to go down the mountain. He wouldn't leave my side until I started trudging down. Then I heard the boom of avalanche blasting and figured he had a point. They knock the snow down before it comes down with its own force, taking everything in its wake.

I figured I made it from 10,535 to 11,500 feet in about an hour. It wasn't too bad.

I spent the rest of my way walking down, which, as I wished I could relay to that ski patroller, seemed a lot more dangerous, because when I was walking up, at least I could see what was coming. When I was walking down, by the time I could hear people, they would have been in striking distance of taking out my knees and their own.

I would have to spend the rest of my time at Top-A-Ten. It gets its name by being at the top of lift 10, and by my estimation, it's about 10,500-feet in elevation.

Top-A-Ten was a flattish section of the mountain designated for cross country skiers and snowshoers. I had discounted Top-A-Ten as not worthy of my training time. I had already passed its altitude. So, when I was looking for an easy hike, I decided to go for Top-A-Ten. It was zero degrees, a through-the-gloves kind of cold, so it ended up being a rough journey after all.

FAT WOMAN ON THE MOUNTAIN

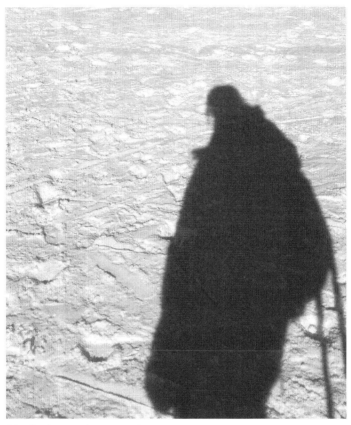

My shadow on the mountain.

I had intended my hike that morning, three miles of wiggling through green and blue trails to get there, to be a warm up. But under the weather conditions, it did nothing but make me colder. The wind whipped at the exposed area of my face. Slivers of my cheeks felt raw and exposed.

As soon as I had reached my destination, where I had planned to do another hour of hiking, I saw a teepee warming area, where showshoers suit up together for group outings. I snuck in, but even though the heater was on, I didn't feel it. I shivered, eating my PB&J (with plum rhubarb jam, thanks to my hosts' collection).

What I wanted more than anything was hot-very hot-chocolate. All I had was water, icy cold water.

Finally, I gave in. It was 10 degrees. The coldest it could be on Kili was minus 25 degrees. This temperature wasn't even close, and I was bailing out, abandoning this hike at least an hour early. Even worse, I decided to download-a term used by ski instructors to refer to taking a chair lift the opposite way, down the mountain.

The chairlift came around, and I was shaky. I was twisted in my poles, and in the moments after I plopped my butt down on the cold seat, my chair was thrust into fast forward, going down. I didn't have the safety bar down, and I was barreling down the mountain. I was afraid to fall and get pierced by a pine. With the chair rocking in the wind, I didn't dare to shimmy myself in place or release my hand from the side. Besides, it felt like it was frozen with frostbite.

I dismounted the chairlift feeling like such a failure.

~~~

My final day of hiking was on Super Bowl Sunday. Instead of sitting around watching the game, I would hit the mountain hard, pushing my way up Galloping Goose.

I decided to spend two hours in High Camp café. I read, wrote in my journal, and watched the skiers saunter in and out, to linger in the thin air as long as I could. After a week of training without doing laundry, my clothing stunk. I was a little uncomfortable letting my scent stew as the other pristine skiers rotated through the tables. But somehow they didn't seem to mind.

Then, a rather friendly group sat next to me and started to chat. They had avalanche shovels on their backpacks. I thought, These are some serious skiers. I asked a woman named Maggie, who had that Telluride sun-kissed skin, where they had been skiing.

She explained that they lived in the town behind the mountain. So when they ski, they hike up the back side of the mountain-with skis on their backs-and ski down the other side. The shovels are for safety since they traverse some treacherous spots along avalanche fields.

These were the first hikers I saw on top of the mountain. I excitedly told them that I, too, had hiked to the top of the mountain to prepare for a Kilimanjaro climb.

As it turned out, Maggie hiked Kilimanjaro the previous year. In fact, she did the same route, the Rongai, and made it all the way to Uhuru peak. That was, after puking at 17,000 feet. The rest of her group cleaned off their lunch table and took turns using the restroom behind High Camp Café.

"You won't believe how slow you'll go," she said. She talked about the sluggish pace that she mimicked with her ski boots on the café's wooden floor. One. Two. One. Two.

It was a bit of a relief, really. I had heard the altitude would make you slower. I certainly was in Telluride, especially in the last leg up to the High Camp Café. Maggie suited up again, zipping up her jacket, and swinging the shovel-heavy backpack back on. She turned to me and said, "Don't worry. You'll make it. And if you don't, it won't matter."

Oh yes, it will, I thought.

8. GETTING THERE

A few minutes before we were supposed to head to the security check at the Amsterdam International Airport, a woman behind me said, "You must be Kara."

I looked up to see what could have been an *Outside* magazine spread. Our trip leader, Ann Gallagher, walked confidently toward the gate with a few climbers in tow.

Amsterdam was the mid-way point for our sixteen-hour journey, and where we would meet our fellow Global Alliance for Africa climbers, who were arriving there via Chicago. Together, we would connect to a KLM flight to Kilimanjaro International Airport.

Chris and I had spent a frustrating hour looking for our traveling companions, approaching youngish travelers sacked out in the otherwise neat airport. They returned blank stares when we asked, "Are you with Global Alliance?"

We were supposed to meet our group in the airport's only McDonalds, but we didn't know their flight was late due to bad weather. We circled around the food court three times and gave up, got a strange European sausage pastry and a cup of coffee so dark that three creams barely made it brown, and headed back to the gate.

Then, the Global Alliance for Africa group found us.

I hoped at least a few of our seven female climbing companions would be at least a little pudgy, needing to drop the ten pounds most people do on a Kili climb, but no such luck. I would be the only fat woman on the mountain.

Ann wore a slick, black, fitted Patagonia down coat. It was ribbed in all the right places. I thought, *Oh, that's what she meant by a light down jacket.*

I had ordered a North Face down jacket from eBay. It was $80, less than half the cost of the same coat I saw when I bought my North Face Summit Series shell. The down jacket was supposed to zip right into the shell, a perfectly-coordinated ensemble.

The eBay deal arrived a week before our trip. It turned out to be a made-in-China fake, synthetic at best, with crooked, embroidered logos. It didn't zip into my jacket but I decided to go with it, even if it made me look puffy and big, like the Michelin Man's bride. It made me sweat.

I only knew Ann over calls and e-mails. She wasn't who I expected. By her phone voice and list of adventures, including the one to come, I was sure she was a fellow thirty-something. She had just turned fifty-two. Ann could have been an Oil of Olay model, with tight, milky skin that only showed a slight bit of creasing around her eyes when she drifted into a short spell of infectious laughter at the end of sentences.

Her husband, who stayed home to tend to their real estate development business, had climbed Mount McKinley, a brutal haul up the tallest mountain in North America. Ann had already climbed Kilimanjaro four times.

This would be her fifth and final trip up Kilimanjaro. Her knees were the only thing stopping her from doing more. She warned they could grow to the size of basketballs by the bottom of the mountain. Still, her vast experience made me glad to have her on our team.

We squeezed in small talk between security checks and bathroom breaks (since we had been pounding several liters of water a day to prevent altitude sickness once the climb arrived).

In the lull of first-meeting chitchat, I remembered the scene from Jon Krakauer's Everest-climbing memoir, *Into Thin Air,* when he sized up his fellow climbers after meeting them the Kathmandu airport. He wrote, "In climbing, having confidence

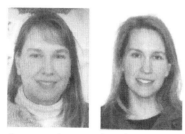

in your partners is no small concern. One climber's actions can affect the welfare of the entire team."

My teammates—Chris, Ann, Sarah, Shawna, Lisa, Lauren, Carla and Karen— seemed slim, trim, and ready for the task. I wondered what

Passport photos a decade apart.

they thought of me. Would I be the one to bring *Into Thin Air*-scale disastrous results to our team? I had to stop thinking about *Into Thin Air.*

I worried I had deceived my group. They had seen photos of me on my website, but most of those were from the waist up. Now, there was no hiding my hips and thighs, which carried the bulk of the fifty pounds I had left to lose. I found myself tugging downward on the Icebreaker merino wool sweater that I bought during last-minute gear shopping mere hours before the flight.

Icebreaker sweaters were all the rage among Telluride ski instructors. I thought my new sweater, coffee-brown with cream trim and zip-up neck, might help me fit in while wearing my size-24 jeans that had grown loose with weight loss. There, in the airport, all my clothes felt tight.

My boots felt heavy and hot. They formed to the contour of my feet through many miles of hiking, so having to buy a new pair at the last minute would have meant a bastion of blisters.

"Hey, we have the same boots," said Sarah, a red-headed assistant guide, while pointing out my Asolo boots, still dusty from practice trails. She flopped herself on the floor and sat cross-legged as she sorted out her gear, at least the lot she carried with her on the plane. "I love your website. I'm so excited to experience this with you," she said. She weighed 120 pounds, the exact amount of weight I lost.

This would be Sarah's second trip up Kilimanjaro. The first time was weeks after her divorce. Angry and determined, she made it to the top despite the sixty-mile-an-hour thrashing winds that could have easily swept her off the mountain's side.

Sarah told me I'd meet the other assistant guide, Shawna, later. Shawna had ventured off to the bathroom. "You can't miss her. She's this tall, gorgeous blonde."

Great, I thought.

Sarah and Shawna's jaunt as assistant guides would test their readiness to lead future Global Alliance for Africa fund-raising climbs. They were best friends who met at their daughters' Montessori school. They first found commonality in their flung-together outfits, while other mothers were primped and poised. Sarah called their clique of two the "Moms Who Don't Shower Club."

I liked Sarah immediately. She had a bookstore but sold her share to be a full-time mother to her two cherub-cheeked children, Pearl and Nell. She carried an 8x10 photo of them with her in a stiff, cardboard envelope that she'd bring to the top of the mountain.

Heads (including my husband's) turned as Shawna approached the group. She was an Uma Thurman-like beauty, movie-star smile and all.

I wanted to hate Shawna. At six-foot-two, she was the tallest blonde on the trip (that's usually my role). She could have been a Patagonia model, showing off her rugged yet fashionable wardrobe. But I couldn't hate her. From the moment we met, she proved to be a wonderful, pure (and yes, drop-dead gorgeous) soul.

Shawna was married to an attorney named Eric. His name alone elicited coos from those who knew him, about his good looks and "honey-do" efficiency and entrepreneurship. He spent the two weeks during her previous Africa absence designing a drying system for Lisa, a fellow climber and artist who rented Shawna and Eric's loft as an art studio.

Shawna was a dichotomy of femininity and force. She cried during sad stories and showed off photos of her six-year-old daughter, Elle.

She was big enough to be a linebacker. I later learned she spent a season playing in a lesbian football league. Same-sex preference was not a requirement to play with the team, though I imagined her teammates wished it was when Shawna joined. Heck, even I thought she was hot.

Though I felt well trained, doubt swept over me when I learned Shawna was one of two climbing companions who had already completed a marathon. The other was Carla, who had done four.

~~~

I had already asked the flight attendant to be placed next to a vacant seat. That way I wouldn't bulge into the person next to me. Chris, who was on the other side of me, was used to being crowded out of his space by my hips.

"Sorry, the flight is full," the attendant replied, perhaps feeling sorry for the soul who would have to squeeze next to me or deal with my hips making the armrests jut up and out of place. My thick thighs and hefty hips are often an annoyance to the person next to me and make it impossible for me to adjust the volume on the in-flight entertainment. (At least I didn't have to ask for a seatbelt extension any more. It can be an awkward moment, flagging down the flight attendant, asking her to hand you the three-foot strap after everyone's eyes were on her for the safety demonstration.)

The Global Alliance for Africa gals were closer to the front of the plane. It was a bit of a relief, actually. Spending eight hours squeezed next to someone who spills over their seat allowance is not the best way to make new friends.

To make matters worse, I was assigned the middle seat. Chris, who had felt my in-flight crunch many times, had the window. I thought about asking for the seat with a view, but didn't want to push the matter with Chris. He was an only child, used to getting his way. Besides, going to Kilimanjaro wasn't his idea. It was mine. Since I was locking him on an airplane for hours on end and dragging him up and down a mountain for six days without a shower, the least I could do was give him the view.

If I were to fight for anything, it would have been the aisle, to let my right leg dangle out, even if it was at risk to get crunched by a cart. But the aisle seat was spoken for. It belonged to Norwegian physician, Petro Aria, one of about thirty doctors on the plane heading to help AIDS patients at Tanzanian hospitals, to climb Kilimanjaro, and, of course, go on safari.

The KLM MD-11 was packed with do-gooders and adventurers. A group of college students was heading for a three-month volunteer stint. A woman behind me was going to an orphanage where thirty-six children live in a family-like setting. She shared her mission with the older couple about to go on safari. They talked about the best places to watch lions tussle with each other like kittens.

Dr. Aria had excused himself from his Kilimanjaro climb, saying he had an injured ankle. I felt sorry for him, having to bow out of the adventure. Yet, part of me wondered how I could injure my ankle in the three days left before the climb. Perhaps Dr. Aria would give me a doctor's note.

Unlike his colleagues who blocked the concession carts while roaming up and down the aisles to chat with the other doctors, he sat alone. He was born in Eritrea, an African country that won its thirty-year fight for independence from Ethiopia. The fight, among many things, was over Eritrea's Red Sea coast. I marked it on the map in my *State of Africa* book with his name. He smiled. I had bought the 752-page tight-print book in the Amsterdam Airport, hoping to learn more about where I was going.

The airplane droned over the Alps, which rose like white waves in Southern Europe. The jagged peaks at Innsbruck, Austria, sat under a blanket of snow. I leaned over Chris's lap, trying to press my face against the glass, wondering how in the world one would climb them. None stood as tall as Kilimanjaro.

The computerized map, with a line showing our route from Europe to Africa, looked like the opening of *Raiders of the Lost Ark*. I looked at it often, with an "Are we there yet?" anxiousness.

The pilot informed us that we'd be flying west of Egypt. The computerized map showed us flying directly over Sudan. When we got there, the Sahara Desert below looked like wrinkled suede.

Chris had calculated our airplane sleep schedule to minimize jet lag. We couldn't afford to start the Kilimanjaro climb, which would begin after two days of visiting Global Alliance for Africa's programs, feeling exhausted.

His plan:

~ Pop a sleeping pill on the Newark to Amsterdam flight. (That worked. It made me snooze about five hours, even as *The Departed* played through my headphones.)

~ Stay awake during the Amsterdam to Kilimanjaro leg so we'd be tired enough to crash once we arrived at night in Africa.

Chris fell asleep three times. He never has trouble sleeping. I do, particularly when I'm nervous or excited about something.

Both emotions were consuming me.

~~~

In between re-reading the hike itinerary on the plane, I started to daydream. I remembered the hours before my return to Camel's Hump. I kept waking up, looking at the clock, turning over and scrunching the pillow under my neck, only to turn over again to check the time. I set the alarm (and checked it a few times) for a 5 a.m. sunrise hike. I wanted to experience the cool, soft air of morning as I braved my way up the mountain. It was supposed to be unusually hot for an early June day in Vermont, maybe 90 degrees, and I didn't want to use the temperature as an excuse for failure.

By night's end, I had accumulated about three hours of sleep. I got up and into my clothes set on the pine chest at the bottom of my bed. I quietly tied my hiking shoes. My pre-packed backpack hung heavy on my shoulder. I quietly left through the front door of my mother's house and was on my way.

What if I had never returned to Camel's Hump? I thought now. *Would I be on this plane?*

~~~

I spent the flight dry-eyed, staring impatiently at the knob fastening my tray table. My legs twitched, antsy because I was used to my daily training schedule-an hour or so on the treadmill or stair stepper, walking around the gym using wide-legged lunge steps, and pushing and pulling on weights, trying to mimic the movements on the mountain.

The pent-up feeling of being on an airplane wasn't sitting well with other passengers either, especially those about to climb Kilimanjaro. They were often out of their seats. They did laps around the aisles, stopping short of the first-class section.

As Dr. Aria slept, I spent an hour trying to figure out a way to gently leave my seat, so as not to stuff my butt in the physician's face as I departed.

While I was up and about, side stepping through the aisles, careful not to belt other people with my hips, I met two friends, who were there to mark their fortieth birthday with an eight-day climb up the Shira Route, which I thought was an awfully long time to go without a shower. I told them I was doing the Rongai Route. I felt them look me up and down.

People paused their circling around the plane aisles for meal, snack and drink breaks, which seemed to happen every hour. Flight attendants pushed large metal cars back and forth, offering a calzone snack or a chicken and orzo pasta dish with salad and a tiramisu-like pudding. They even set up candy bar snacks near their kitchen area in the back. My favorite part was the final snack: ice cream. It came in a little cup with one of those cute wooden spoons.

My neck craned back, looking for the next round of meals. I ate everything given to me. I wondered if I was eating out of boredom or fear.

No, I was finally legitimately carbo-loading.

9. GROUND LEVEL

As we wove our way through the mud-caked walls and rusty tin roof shack maze of an Arusha slum, kids appeared from the corner following us, as if we were all part of a parade. The ground was a reddish mud, with ditches carved by the rains.

We were there to see Global Alliance for Africa's tap program. The tap partnership with the Msamaria Orphans program allows a co-op of about fifteen families to buy a tap into the city's municipal water program. Global Alliance for Africa picks up the $400 cost. After all, that's more than the annual income of most families we visited.

I talked with some women about how the tap-a plain brass spigot unlike our fancy, nickel-plated, "must-have" hardware from Home Depot-changed their lives. They now had water to drink, as well as to prepare food and bathe their children-many of whom were not their own, but AIDS orphans they support alongside their own kids. Also, the women could sell the water at an affordable price to their neighbors.

The women explained today would not be a good day for business because it was going to rain. *Oh my God*, I thought. *These people depend on the rain for water. Water to drink! What if it doesn't rain? And I was worried about being away from a*

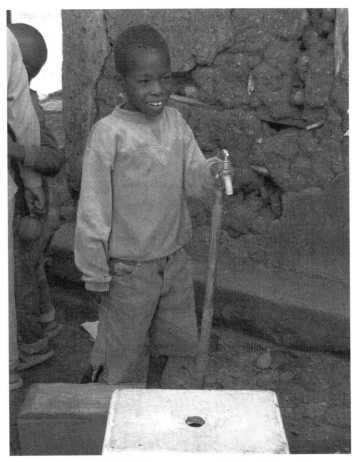

An adorable boy I met while visiting one of Global Alliance for Africa's water tap programs.

shower for a week.

I continued to talk with the women, while a little guy clung to his mother's leg. It was snug in the square where the family hung laundry and hosted the tap. Some of our traveling companions went back out into an open area, where they were surrounded by children.

I remembered Shawna talked about how tough it was to find Polaroid camera film earlier in the trip. In the days of digital images, I wondered what kind of retro project the artist was planning.

Then, I saw Shawna squatting down, like a catcher, with the Polaroid camera in her mitts. She was eye-to-eye with the kids, as she took each of their pictures and gave it to them.

They didn't speak English. She didn't speak Swahili. Somehow the international language of "I'm next!" worked well. The kids lined up, striking a pose for the camera. Some were gleeful, smiling wide, as Shawna captured their happiness. Others looked shell-shocked, with a blank stare into the camera. One held a teddy bear by the leg, and seemed to wonder what the heck Shawna was doing getting in so close. He sprinted off to show someone when he saw his image develop.

I smiled at the goodness of the moment, an instant gratification gesture to give them a photo of themselves. It was a rarity compared to our capture-everything-society. I wondered how many of the kids were orphans.

After three days of seeing the Global Alliance for Africa programs we supported, I felt a mixed bag of dread and hope. I knew my fund-raising effort, $12,000, would do a lot of good, but there was so much work to do.

Tom Derdak, Global Alliance for Africa's director, held a debriefing, a surreal sort of meeting at a Chinese restaurant where we emptied out our guilt of how we live, compared to the lives of most people in Tanzania. I felt guilty eating a meal out when the per capita income there is about $600.

Carla asked, "What's the one most important thing we can do?"

Tom responded, "Tell people about Africa."

~~~

We were swept off to our climb by bus. It would take about four hours to get to Kibo Hotel, a popular base camp for Kili climbers.

We didn't have much time between offloading the bus, which had been stacked high with our roped-down bags, and our pre-climb briefing. So we set our stuff down in our rooms and headed to the restaurant.

I was the only one who didn't order a beer. I had read alcohol hinders acclimatization, so I decided I would wait to have one until I was down the mountain. I wanted one, though, after our African Walking Company trip coordinator told us, "If you vomit more than five times near the summit, you need to come down. We want to return you to the bottom with a pulse."

The afternoon meeting was held at a long table in the Kibo Hotel restaurant. Its walls were lined with Sharpie-signed shirts of successful Kilimanjaro climbers. Though a few windows were open, it felt warm and stuffy in the room. Or maybe that was just anxiety, making it tough to breathe.

The coordinator reviewed a hand-drawn map, which couldn't possibly have been to scale with its squiggly lines up to the summit. It looked like it was sketched on the back of a paper placemat in a restaurant. Still, it did a nice job detailing how many hours it would take to get from point to point. But by then, I had already memorized the itinerary. I had marked it on my wall calendar and my pocket calendar. Even though each leg was an hour later than originally set forth, I was surprised when some of our climbers seemed wowed at the brutal haul ahead of us. Carla and Karen gasped at the pre-climb play by play.

Carla and Karen grew up together in blue-collar Chicago. They became best friends in Catholic high school, where Karen had to work after school to fund her tuition. Karen, a short, Italian woman with the muscles of Madonna, had run a nursing referral company. Carla was a tall, thin woman who worked in public relations. They set each other on fire with laughter over the smallest things. They both had been married, and right around the time of the Kilimanjaro climb both were in the middle of a divorce. For them, finding and signing up for this climb was coincidence.

Carla's friend was in the market for a new home in fall 2006. They heard about a stylish, eco-friendly development in Miller Beach, Indiana, about forty-five minutes outside Chicago. The developer of the project happened to be Ann, our climb leader, who was showing the model that day.

Ann got to talking with Carla and mentioned the upcoming trip to Africa. With the housing slump in full force, Ann didn't sell the condo to Carla's boyfriend. However, Carla was sold on the trip.

Carla then called Karen, as she did with most things. "So, I was thinking about climbing Kilimanjaro. It's a fund raiser for AIDS orphans. Do you want to come along?"

"Uh, okay."

And so it was done. While both women were in terrific shape, Carla a marathoner and Karen an avid walker and power yogi, when it came to mountain climbing they were out of their element.

At the base of the mountain, our trip coordinator looked confused when Carla said, "So, when does the pep talk come in?"

Our group laughed nervously. Ann, who had been smiling and nodding along with the description of the road ahead, chimed in, "She's wondering if you could say something like, 'You can do it!'"

He didn't oblige. Instead, he reviewed the map again and said most people who are in shape will find the first four days strenuous but do-able. Nevertheless some people, no matter how well trained they are, get sick, very sick, and have to turn back a couple of days into the journey. Most people who give up do so on summit day, right about Hans Meyer Cave, a few hours from Uhuru Peak.

"In the beginning, you are excited. But then, around Jamaica Rocks, you start to get tired. It's dark. You are cold, frustrated, and want to turn around. You need a faithful heart, and a strong mind," he said. "*Pole, pole*, and you'll get there."

"Pole, pole" is Swahili for "slowly, slowly." The slower you hike the mountain, the better you will acclimatize. When I first heard that the slowest hikers have the best chances of reaching the summit, I thought, *Now that's my kind of mountain. I can compete in this game.*

The coordinator dismissed us from the restaurant, saying we'd need to be ready at 8 a.m. We needed to be ready with a duffle bag of our supplies, weighing no more than fifteen kilograms, about thirty-three pounds.

We headed back to our hotel rooms. The rooms were connected by a covered, open-air hallway facing a garden. The flowers, red and fuchsia, reminded Karen of Maui where she once owned a farm.

The easy-going setting of the hotel made me want to meander, especially after four days of travel from one end to the globe to the other, and then some. As a bus rolled up, with the clamor of climbers who just came down the mountain, I was reminded there was much work to do. People who returned from the climb headed straight to the shower, then walked stiff-legged to the lobby for a beer. They eased into chairs around a central fireplace and encouraged those coming in for the climb that they, too, could do it.Chris and I headed back to Room Number 8 and unlocked the door with a key attached to a gigantic piece of wood.

Ann took it upon herself to go to each room with an old-fashioned hand-held scale to make sure each bag was within the weight limit. Something about scales always makes me nervous. She had a couple rooms to go before she got to ours.

I wanted to make excuses for my bag, as I looked at the puckered green duffel bag. *Of course it weighs more. I'm a big gal, my clothes are bigger, heavier.* Or, *I'm the one toting all the emergency stuff that Chris couldn't be bothered with.*

I was certain it weighed more than fifteen kilograms. It took my father-in-law, an organizational genius, to get everything in the Army surplus bag.

I unlatched the black metal buckle and frantically started to pull things out of my bag. The first aid kit could go, because I knew there would be at least three on the backs of our guides and Ann. I moved onto the toiletries, which I thought I had twice as much as I needed. I even took out a couple rolls of toilet paper, fearing that would be what would break my porter's back.

Then, I hit my hard candy collection. One of our former Kilimanjaro climber consultants suggested bringing it to suck in the dry air that comes near the top of the mountain. Another said we'd want to have some to give to kids who wait along the path. No need to convince me, one reason would have been enough.

I had brought three bags of candy: a bag of Lifesavers, a package of root beer barrels, and an assorted mega-size one that I'd already broken into. Now, looking at the five pounds of candy, I realized this was beyond excessive. A butterscotch disk (my third since returning to the room, perhaps to calm my nervousness) melted in my mouth as I removed the root beer barrels and assorted candies from my backpack. I didn't throw them away, just moved them into a bag that wouldn't go up the mountain. I figured I needed the Lifesavers the most. They just sounded like the best option.

Ann was getting closer. I could hear her in the hotel room next door. I heard Carla howl with laughter as Karen refused to deplete her snack supplies. Karen brought Pringles because the chips wouldn't crush in the can and two pounds of hiker's chocolate, the kind that wouldn't melt in the African sun. Note to self: *Make friends with Karen.*

I swiftly stuffed my remaining items back into place as Ann knocked on our door. She reported that everyone else's bags had weighed in okay. We were last. I dragged my duffle bag off the bed and hooked it onto the scale.

Chris's biceps bulged as he held both the scale and my bag in the air. "Fourteen kilos." Chris's turn: "Thirteen kilos."

Of course, Chris's bag weighed less than mine.

The dinner that night was a buffet. It wasn't the sort of thing I would want as a last meal. I thought I better eat up so I would have plenty of energy to get up the mountain and back down again. I could eat something better later. There were lots of carbs-rice, potatoes and bread, some kind of spicy chicken dish, eggplant something-or-other, and a beef stew. I took a little bit of each before returning to the table, where the first-time climbers sat pie-eyed over the five-day haul ahead.

Karen finally admitted what most of us thought. "I'm terrified."

Others, including me, nodded in agreement.

"Aw, guys, don't worry about it, you'll do great," Ann said. It wasn't all that comforting, knowing on each of her ascents at least two people didn't make it up the mountain.

Finally Shawna reminded the group, "Remember, you're not climbing the summit tomorrow. Tomorrow is just a hike. Each day is just a hike, making you stronger for the summit. Then, when summit day comes, you are really ready."

It was as though the air returned to the table, and we could all exhale. I swear I heard a collective sigh. That's what we needed to hear. To break it down, bit by bit.

No, I never climbed a mountain so big, but I have done lots of long, strenuous day hikes, some several days in a row. Yes, on summit day, I would be ready, I told myself, gnawing on a bit of beef stew.

The rest of the dinner focused on other people's fears about the journey.

I talked about my mother, who in the days before my flight to Africa, reminded me, "Be careful up there," in the months before I climbed. "I worry. I'm your mother."

"I know, Mom. I know. But I'll be fine."

"You're going with guides, right?" Of course she knew the answer to this was "yes." I had already told her several times.

She and my step-father bought a traveler's guide to Tanzania and worried even more when they couldn't find my route, the Rongai route, in the Kilimanjaro section.

They had a right to be concerned. This time my older brother wouldn't be available to pick me up if I went down the wrong side of the mountain (like Chris and I did on Mount Mansfield).

In December, as my hike approached, people really got paranoid.

As I arrived at work one day, my *Courier News* colleague Angela, who rarely ventured into New York City even though she lived a thirty-minute train ride away, announced, "You can't go up that mountain. I'm a mother and I worry. I'm not going to stop worrying until you get back here."

I looked up at the wall-mounted television in our newsroom, where we play CNN constantly, and understood what Angela was talking about.

There was a constant stream of news about three missing ice climbers who went out to conquer Mount Hood, but were barraged by bad—no, horrific—blinding snow storms. After they reached the mountain's summit on December 8, Kelly James, 48, of Texas, injured his arm. His friends—Brian Hall, 37, also of Dallas; and Jerry "Nikko" Cooke, 26, of New York City—went to get help.

The unrelenting weather hindered the search for James, Hall and Cooke—all experienced climbers-whose journey had gone awry. James's body was found a few days later, hunkered in a snow cave, where he called his family to tell them he was hurt and Cooke and Hall had gone for help.

Each day during the search one of my family members or friends would e-mail or call to check in, and say, "Oh, by the way, did you hear about those missing climbers on Mount Hood?"

Each time, I had to explain that climbing Mount Hood is much more treacherous terrain. I wasn't rock climbing to the top of Kilimanjaro, I was "walking." That usually worked in calming their nerves. But each mention of the Mount Hood ordeal stressed me out a bit more than I liked.

I explained this around the dinner table, and my climbing companions nodded as if they had similar conversations. Their friends and family had also brought up the Mount Hood climb, and they had to feign courage and convince them all would be well on our mountain climb.

Kilimanjaro was a completely different type of climb, on completely different terrain. And not to worry. *We were worried enough.*

Lauren, a climber in our group who lived and breathed extreme sports, may not have been worried. When it came to Kilimanjaro, Lauren thought, "Bring it on."

Lauren grew up in Utah with Samantha Dwyer, one of Global Alliance for Africa's few U.S.-based employees. Samantha had climbed Kilimanjaro in 2006, and when she told Lauren about it, Lauren was so moved by her friend's experience, she signed up for the next year.

At age twenty-three, Lauren was the youngest climber in our group. She worked at a heli-ski operation at Snowbird Ski resort and took advantage of discounted extreme skiing whenever she could, even with a shattered kneecap. Lauren learned about the injury while playing rugby for a semi-professional woman's league. She decided to finish out the season rather than get it fixed. Two years later, it still wasn't fixed.

Lauren had already decided climbing Kilimanjaro would be a fine way to leave this world. She was young, but had already decided that she wanted her death to be by adventure.

"I want it to be the kind of thing people talk about like, 'Did you hear about Lauren? Yo, she got mauled by a bear!'"

I could only respect her for that. As a newspaper reporter I saw death was everywhere, especially when it's not expected. I've written about a guy killed when the tree he was chopping landed on him. A grandmother was crushed, with her grandson in the car, when her SUV that she had stopped on the side of the highway because of car trouble rolled on top of her. Death doesn't have to be so freakish. People die every day doing the mundane-driving to work, walking across the street. You just never know when it's going to happen.

So why not take chances and do the things I wanted to do? I was going to die eventually. Why not here and now, having fun?

10. DAY 1: *"POLE, POLE"*

We dragged our luggage like super-sized sacks of potatoes to a parking lot, next to a lush garden of red and yellow flowers. Our guides tossed our luggage on the top of two Range Rovers like pillows. They were packed high and roped tight to the top of the vehicles.

While our guides gathered our lunches for the day and an assortment of supplies including water barrels, we stood under the shade of a Kibo Hotel overhang and felt a dense heat that permeated the shade. I could feel sweat bubbling up under my sunscreen.

Chris snapped a photo of us waiting there. I wore a bandana around my head and a breathable baby-blue top. I smiled wide for the photo. We looked ready for the mountain, but we weren't quite there yet.

Most people stay at Kibo Hotel because it is close to the mountain, about fifteen minutes away from the base of the Marangu Route. The Marangu Route, also known as the Coca-Cola route (because you can buy soda and beer on the way up) is the most popular. It takes four days to climb, as opposed to our five, giving people less time to acclimatize. Hence, their chance of summit success is lower.

We were driving to the other side of the mountain, the Kenya side. It would be a bumpy two-hour journey passing through villages. Women trudged down the water-worn roads of red earth, carrying giant bushels of bananas on their heads. Kids ran alongside the bus and waved.

When we arrived in Moru Village, we were far away from commercial centers. The hill was above wooden shacks, on a plateau that seemed to go on forever. We slathered ourselves with sunscreen—something we would have to do every hour on the mountain—as we were hiking just 200 miles from the equator.

We gathered in a circle to sign the guestbook, a marker of who had been along the trail. Meanwhile, our porters huddled around our gigantic pile of bags and equipment, including my bulging duffle.

As mine was assigned to a porter, Sampson, I said, "Samahani"—Swahili for "Sorry."

It didn't feel right having someone else carry my load. I knew the brunt of carrying just two day's worth of gear from our Grand Canyon journey, and it was hard, really hard, hiking up with a gigantic load on your back.

I had been told being a porter in Tanzania is a job, a good job. It's back-breaking work for sure. But, Sarah explained, the porters are acclimatized and strong. We leave an hour before they do, and they zoom right past and arrive an hour before we do.

"It's amazing," Sarah told me.

During the previous year's climb, Samantha, one of Global Alliance for Africa's state-side employees, felt it wasn't right to have other people carry her nearly forty-pound back pack. She decided to do it herself. Then, three days into the climb, she couldn't carry it herself anymore, and there wasn't a porter assigned to her bag. So Tom, Global Alliance for Africa's director, took over the task. While the big bag doesn't go up with climbers on Summit night, Tom didn't summit, but Sam did.

We were introduced to the top staff members—Meke (the chief guide), Robbie and Lasti (the assistant guides), James (the head porter), and Trophine (the cook).

Then, without ceremony, it was time to start walking. The trailhead on the Rongai route has a large wooden sign with the following guidelines.

Points to remember:
1. *Hikers attempting to reach the summit should be physically fit.*
2. *If you have a sore throat, a cold, or breathing problems, do not go beyond 3,000 meters above sea level.*
3. *Children under ten years of age are not allowed above 3,000 meters above sea level.*
4. *If you have heart or lung problems do not attempt the mountain at all without consulting your doctor.*
5. *Allow plenty of time for the body to acclimatize by ascending slowly.*
6. *Drink four to five liters of fluid each day. Water is best, but fruit juices are a good supplement.*
7. *If symptoms of mountain sickness or high altitude diseases persist, please descend immediately and seek medical treatment. Our rescue team is always alert to rescue casualties at Kibo, Horombo and Kinapa H/Q.*
8. *Please avoid wild fires by not throwing burning cigarettes butts when ascending and descending.*
9. *Please leave the mountain as clean as you found it.*

As we started the Rongai Route, I thrust my poles into the red equatorial soil like an Olympic cross country skier. My pace was strong and powerful—like my final training hikes in the backwoods of New Jersey. Chris and I only managed a few vigorous strides on the path before Robbie, an assistant guide, called out: "*Pole, pole.*"

It was the mantra for the wedding march-like pace needed to make it to the top of the mountain. Our climb began at an altitude higher than Denver, Mile High City.

Climbers must go slowly every step of the way to avoid altitude sickness, which can cause massive headaches, nausea, and, in the worst cases, death.

At first I wondered if I could stand the lethargy of it. Later, I wondered if I could keep up. Aside from the soil and the surroundings, the trail felt like the others I had been on in New Jersey. A gradual ascent, but nothing I couldn't handle. Then, as we came to a grove with a hut, the children we met came to the trail with outstretched hands saying, "Chocolate. Chocolate."

I got a sense this happened every time hikers passed, so I pulled mine out of my bag and handed it over. I wondered if I would have done that in my heavier days. Now it wasn't about the snacks in my bags, it was about the journey. It felt good to set my chocolate free.

We continued on until we came to a grove of trees. There was an outhouse, but judging from the smell twenty feet away, it seemed like a bad idea to use it. Most of us settled to squat behind it, rather than dare open the door to find what was inside.

It felt nice to rest, but I wasn't all that tired. We pulled out our boxed lunch—buttered bread, an orange that was green, and a juice box. One of the keys of hiking in high altitude is staying well hydrated—five liters a day. So when you weren't walking, you should be drinking. I took some time to chug.

The truth was this felt easy, familiar. I had been on a hike like this before. I started to gush with self-confidence, there in the grove.

A few minutes after we stopped, the porters passed us. I let out a cheerful, "Jambo" (Swahili for hello) to each one as they lugged our stuff on their heads.

We picked up our daypacks-which had the essentials from sunhats to water-and started on through the rainforest. It had been overcast all day. Then, I realized, even on the trail, I had yet to see Kilimanjaro's peak.

Although I had seen pictures, I didn't really know what to expect on the journey up Mount Kilimanjaro. We were walking toward the peak, without seeing what we were in for. Maybe that was a good thing.

As you reach the summit, the conditions make it difficult for plants—and humans—to survive. Hiking Mount Kilimanjaro is like hiking up the side of the globe. At the bottom you are in the farmer's fields, just south of the equator. The temperature drops a bit with each step up the mountain as you hike through five ecological zones. The lower mountain forest has a cool rich climate. The volcanic soil is fertile for growing, and home to elderberry, raspberry, and begonias. Every once in a while you can spot an Impatiens Kilimanjari-an orange-red flower that can be found nowhere else in the world. From there, you reach the upper mountain forest with lichens, mosses, and ferns growing on trees. Birds are often seen there.

As you approach the heather and moorland section of the mountain, the height of the trees starts to shrink. The sky above opens from the lack of the canopy of trees. Instead, there are giant senecios, a prehistoric-looking plant that looks like part cactus and part palm tree, and flowering lobelia plants. Above 13,000 feet you reach the alpine desert where the dry, thin air makes it summer every day and winter every night. There isn't much plant life at all, as the conditions make it difficult for anything to grow.

Then at last you reach the summit. With its glaciers—what little there are left of them—it is like standing on the arctic high above the tropics. The glaciers are really one of the reasons to go up this mountain soon, to see them before they are gone. At one time, most of Kilimanjaro was covered with an ice cap a hundred meters deep. Now only a fraction remains. It could be gone within the next half century.

Another quick break and we reached camp one—a lovely little grove. The porters had already set up the campground and were cooking dinner. The smell of soup wafted through the campground.

I put my backpack down. After three hours of hiking, I was a little tired but I felt good. I pushed myself into the tent. At six-feet tall, I never have handled this gracefully. I normally get caught up in a rope or slide down on my sleeping bag. As we lay there, having a little rest before tea, I thought, This will be my home for the next week.

I kind of liked being detached from the world, knowing there was just a bit of nylon separating me from the elements and that everything I needed could fit in a duffle bag. It felt free.

Despite this feeling of meager existence, we had so much stuff in the duffle bags that it was hard not having it fall out every time we looked for something. A friend had told me to pack everything in labeled plastic bags to help when I got more disoriented further up the mountain. It didn't seem to help.

Every time I unpacked my bag, it made a great big mess.

We are indeed creatures of habit. Chris and I automatically picked sides of the tent, matching the sides we slept on in our own bed. Just as I started to settle down, there was a call out that "washy-washy" water was outside our tents.

Since we were going without a shower for so long, the porters prepared a pan of water that went from warm to cold in a matter of minutes so we could stay somewhat hygienic throughout the journey. I never knew how tough it could be to take a sponge bath sitting down in the alcove of my tent.

I didn't dare stand up and take mine outside with so many guys around. I didn't want to be laughed at. I still felt—and was—jiggle-y, bumpy, and very unsure of my own body. I didn't like being in a bathing suit around anyone, including my husband.

After thirty minutes of trying to wash up without standing up, it was time for tea. So I tried to neatly pack my things in my bag and backed out of my tent, nearly tripping on the cord to get out. I laughed a little at myself, about to let out a few words of self-deprecating humor, when I brushed my hair out of my face and looked up.

There it was: the peak of Mount Kilimanjaro.

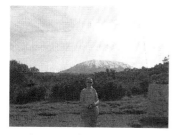
My first view of Mount Kilimanjaro.

I gasped at its beauty. It was so magnificent, so wondrous, and so very, very high.

It was an awesome force of nature pointing through the clouds. It was better than any photograph I had seen.

It was imposing, and seemed like it was miles and

miles away. It was.

Meke said it had just snowed, which was good because it would be hard packed by the time we were on it-four days from then. The snow seemed unreal because I was sweating.

After some tea time, it was time to take an acclimatization hike. One strategy in hiking in high altitudes is to climb high and sleep low. In other words, push your body a little higher to experience that new altitude, and come back down.

By now, we had gotten to know each other, and had taken on the tradition of giving each other mountain nicknames, something that characterized the kind of hiker we were or hoped to be.

Mama Kubwa was my Swahili nickname for the climb. It meant "Big Woman." We all had nicknames. Some were given. Meke called Chris "Papa Impala" because he was the only male climber, and impalas have many wives. Some were requested. Our trip coordinator Ann was "Mama Kiongosi," meaning Boss Woman.

I didn't mind Mama Kubwa. I made it my battle cry up the mountain. Fat was what set me apart from the other climbers. But instead of holding me back, as it did for many years, it was what moved me forward.

As the sun set behind the mountain, the air grew crisp. I had been in hiking pants and short sleeves all day. When it came time for dinner, it was time to put on my fleece jacket.

James arrived with wonderful vegetable soup, and a platter of "Tilapia from Lake Victoria," he announced. We later wondered, does Lake Victoria even have that kind of fish—and how on earth did they get it here on the mountain? It would be the first of wonderfully surprising meals on the mountain.

My fellow trekkers and I laughed our way through the

dinner. Meke came in to see how we were all feeling and to give us details about the next day's seven-hour journey up to Kikelewa Cave-about 11,000 feet above sea level. We would walk our way "*pole, pole*" to lunch, seeing caves and giant senecios along the way, and finish at the campground.

During the evening briefing, we asked Meke what the weather would be like the next day.

"It will be unpredictable," he said, knowing he was exactly right.

FAT WOMAN ON THE MOUNTAIN

11. THE LONG HAUL

I slept, but not well. I went to sleep wearing a full set of long underwear just because I had it and it felt outdoorsy. Ten minutes into zipping up my winter-grade sleeping bag, I was sweating. Chris had already fallen asleep by the time I yanked the long underwear off and decided to doze in what I did at home—T-shirt and panties.

I spent a half hour, sometime in the middle of the night, wondering how to best maneuver my way to my bathroom bucket, which sat in what would be the foyer of our tent. Finally I woke Chris up anyway as I fumbled around, and sometimes swore. But he went back to bed and I would be awake for another half hour or so remembering how Meke said villagers might sneak into our camp, and by the way, lions might, too. Perhaps they were kidding about the lions, but I wasn't going to take them lightly. Didn't Hemingway write about a leopard that ventured much farther up the mountain?

I awoke at about 6 a.m., hearing the dawn rustle of the staffers, preparing for our next meal and our next move.

The foam mattresses, a $25 rental, kept us somewhat comfortable through the night. Though calling them "mattresses" went a little too far. Or maybe I was just sore from our first day on the mountain.

Each morning, our official wakeup call would be a staff member zipping our tent open and asking about how we slept, how we felt, and what we would like to drink.

As always, they brought tea with milk and sugar. There was something so warm and comforting about red African tea. I didn't drink it at home, but there on the mountain, it made me feel at home.

I was sitting up, still enveloped in a sleeping bag that I was glad to be able to fit in, when Chris chimed, "Happy Valentine's Day!"

I echoed, "Happy Valentine's Day!" I turned to give him a kiss while one arm reached into my bag to pull out his gift, about a dozen heart-shaped lollipops, figuring they would help him in the days of dry air ahead. I put them in a shiny, red bag.

I opened my card from Chris, which had a picture of Charlie Brown on the front. Charlie Brown held a gigantic paintbrush, trying to get a stack of Valentines just right. Snoopy, who was by his side, looked frazzled, with his ears upright.

On the front it read, "I was trying to make you the perfect Valentine..."

On the inside, it said, "But then I realized you were the perfect Valentine."

He signed it, "Love, Chris."

He handed me a Walgreens bag with gifts: a notebook with a cat following a heart on a string and two Valentine's Day puzzles, which came in the boxes much like individually-sized conversation hearts. One, when complete, said, "Be mine."

I was already gushing, embarrassed that I only bothered to bring lollipops that I suggested he share with our fellow climbers. Then, he pulled a necklace from his bag. It was a string of small black beads, with a carved elephant in the middle. He had picked it up from the Kibo Hotel gift shop while I was still fiddling with my luggage.

I was on the brink of tears. It was an amazingly thoughtful gesture from the love of my life, who has been known to pick up my valentines on February 13, digging through what's left in the local drug store. This time, he thought ahead, before border crossings, before the onslaught of pre-Valentine's Day commercials. Perhaps he knew that if ever there was a time when I needed encouragement and love, it would be now.

I tucked the puzzles in my backpack for entertainment in the downtime to come. I fastened the necklace around my neck. It was the perfect accessory to wear the rest of the way up the mountain.

We took turns using the water for "washy-washy," which had grown a bit cold in our romantic interlude. The in-tent sponge bath, on the other hand, was not in the least bit sexy, trying to erase the smells from the day before.

I tried to dress quickly but it seemed everything that I needed had drifted to the bottom of my duffle bag. So, the contents of my once neatly-organized bag were scattered on my side of the tent, infringing on Chris' territory. Breakfast was starting soon, so I tried to get everything back in order, putting all the things I'd need for the last, coldest days on the bottom, and shoving everything else on top.

Chris had already moved to stuffing his sleeping bag into the compression bag. I wasn't even completely dressed. Pulling pants on while horizontal is not easy, but it was easier when Chris left and I had the entire tent to thrash around in as I, too, tried to get my sleeping bag in the compression bag.

It started well. The sack seemed like it was designed to fit one-quarter of the sleeping bag. After that, it was a wrestling match and the sleeping bag was winning. I'd punch the blue bag into the sack, while other parts of the overstuffed blanket would spill out. Again and again, I squeezed the blanket in the bag, making miniscule progress with each sweaty maneuver. It was hard to tell if it was the altitude or my attitude that was making it so difficult.

Since Chris had already packed, he left the tent to give me some space. He was the only man on the hike, and he decided that he would share his heart-shaped lollipops with the fellow climbers, drawing a collective "Aw." He handed the candies to the porters, who seemed perplexed that a man was giving them sweets and explaining this holiday about love.

Chris came back to the tent. His bag of candy was nearly empty. "We need to get going. It's time for breakfast."

I showed my sleeping bag progress to Chris. The bag was almost in, but was hanging messily out of the edge. With a few swift pushes, Chris completed the job, and helped me carry everything to the pile of other climbers' bags, ready to go up the mountain.

Breakfast had already begun when we arrived. I set our malaria pills, gingko biloba, and Airborne tablets in front of us. We each got fruit, toast, and a fried egg. We were encouraged to eat. Day two would be a long one.

It was a seven-hour hike, with a vertical rise of 3,280 feet. It wasn't the steepest of our days, but nonetheless it was a long haul.

But I felt good, well prepared. Day one and its barely three hour walk was like a warm up, and this seven-hour day was just like any of the practice hikes that we'd been on. I kept doing the math in my head. I had walked seven hours plenty of times. I reminded myself that this was no longer than Camel's Hump

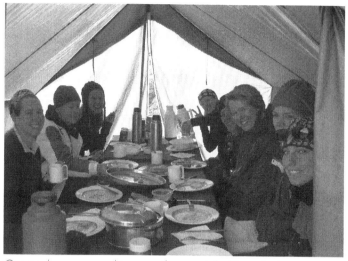

Our meals were served to us up the mountain. The only thing we needed to worry about was walking.

and I could do that.

It's normally clear in the morning at Moorland Camp before the afternoon clouds roll in. The landscape stretched out in front of me, Mawenzi's jagged peak to the left, Kilimanjaro's square top to the right.

Seeing our target, our destination, it finally felt like I was on my way there. My heart swooned, thinking that I was finally doing this. No more blather about how I'm going to climb Kilimanjaro. I was there.

But though Kilimanjaro was there, beckoning me, it did seem far away. I was never great at judging distances, but it felt like starting a mountain climb two towns away from the base of the mountain. First we'd have to swoop over to the base of Mawenzi, before traversing the saddle between the two peaks. It was far away and the only way to get there was on foot. White butterflies fluttered around us on our way up the mountain.

I was feeling really good. An hour into the ascent, we took a break at what the guides called a cave, though it felt little more than an overhang. Still, it was enough to give us fair-skin climbers shade. Lisa re-braided her long blond hair. Karen pulled the ear plugs out of her ears and said she was listening to music because she was afraid of the sound of her breathing, which was far heavier than when she walked in the Chicago area.

Someone talked about a woman who was killed while jogging and wearing an iPod in Chicago. Apparently, she didn't hear the dump truck coming that was about to run her over.

Sure, my breathing was heavier, but it was something I had expected. I would have worried if it wasn't that way.

Meke ordered us to drink water at the break. Lots of it. With all of the water and some people who had already taken Diamox, a drug designed to help people shed fluids (as in pee it out), there were plenty of pit stops. At a spot behind a yellow-flowered bush, I discovered my "monthly friend" came along for the trip. It was early. Altitude and athletic stress has been known to do strange things to a woman's body. Like I needed cramps along with altitude sickness! Luckily, I had supplies to handle the situation.

From that point forward, the existing outhouses were putrid. We had a toilet tent, but that was only where we set up camp. For the journey in between, it was a matter of peeing in places somewhat out of view of the rest of the group. Though with each pit stop, there seemed to be less and less modesty.

Global Alliance for Africa had selected the company—African Walking Company—we climbed with. As we approached the Second Rongai Cave, I realized we were incredibly spoiled. We approached and saw a table set up inside.

Napkins were folded in glasses, like the wings of our butterfly companions. Our chef Trophine and a few other members of the mountain staff huddled around a stove where a carrot soup was just about finished.

Trophine, who didn't speak much English (which may have explained his painful shyness), never had any formal training as a chef. But Meke said he was a natural, having learned everything he knew about cooking over gas stoves in the wild. One taste of his soups and we learned Trophine had a gift.

They had gathered up their best team for us, knowing our climb was all about giving back to Africa.

James brought out corn bread, and then a platter of fanciful salad. Carrots, red pepper, and avocado topped the lettuce. He sprinkled a lime dressing on top. It was a happy little lunch, and out in the wild it felt downright gourmet. We sat there and wowed at the culinary endeavor at about 10,500 feet above sea level, far away from any kind of traditional kitchen.

I stretched my hamstring, pulling my heel to my butt, and pushed my hands to the ground. After four hours of hiking, I was feeling it. I wasn't sore. I was just worn.

The beautiful blue day was starting to look more gray, as the afternoon clouds started making their appearance on the horizon. Then, as the sky promised, it started to rain.

Normally, this would be the point of a hike when I would turn back to head to my car and call it a day. I would spend the evening with a warm cup of tea in fuzzy pajama pants. But I was on the mountain now. Even if the rest of the trek was a torrential downpour, it was my time to be there. I had to trudge on through the clouds, which were a lot closer to me than on ground level. Some low clouds brushed through the terrain and over us as we continued on our path up the mountain.

I pulled on a poncho so my bag wouldn't get wet. But it ripped as I slipped it over my head, leaving a gaping hole. (When I returned home, I'd realize one of the features of my bag was a rain cover, found in a bottom compartment. Oops.) It was so important to stay dry. If it was going to be a rainy week on the mountain, once wet your things would never feel dry.

Karen was not feeling well. We stopped often to allow her to keep up. Meke wanted to keep the group together. Besides, we were in no hurry. The only thing we had to do that day was hike—through the drizzle.

We arrived at camp, and Chris practically dove in the tent. His head was pounding with a headache, his stomach swirled like a whirlpool. It was time for a dose of Diamox. Chris is normally averse to taking medications. He was more likely to let a cold drag out instead of popping medication. So I was glad he easily surrendered to taking the medication.

I was compelled to hold him, sit with him, and say that all would be well, he would be well. But each word out of my mouth was piercing, not soothing. He demanded to be alone. I went to the mess tent, where Chris was missing his tea and popcorn time. I had some time to bond with just the girls. But in my mind I worried about Chris.

It was only day two, and he felt sick. What if the Diamox didn't work, and he'd have to turn back? Before the climb we decided that if one of us wasn't well enough to continue on, the other should at least try to summit. Still, I didn't want to make that choice.

By the time we reached the camp, the clouds had burned off, leaving a bright blue sky above. From the cloud line, Kenya looked like a green agricultural quilt, the kind of patchwork view one would need an airplane to see. I took wobbly steps. My legs felt the strain of our seven-hour march. I teetered between volcanic pebbles from the edge of Kikelewa Caves Camp back to my tent.

At 11,811 feet, I was higher than I've ever climbed, with three days and more than 7,000 feet to go. I felt strong, but everyone around me was starting to feel sick.

FAT WOMAN ON THE MOUNTAIN

12. MOUNTAIN MADNESS

From my vantage point above the world, I realized I was in a different realm. I was seeing things I never thought possible. I was pushing my body harder than ever before. I was working through things even when it felt uncomfortable to do so.

Sometimes I think that is the trouble with losing weight. We can use food to ease difficult situations and feel comfortable. To change, we often need to feel uncomfortable. It is so easy to fall back on old patterns even if you have good intentions.

After resting and staying put, Chris started to feel better. He rejoined the group at dinner. I could tell he was dragging, but at least he was upright.

The next morning brought beautiful weather and most people were feeling better as their bodies adjusted to the new altitude. That was, except for Karen and Carla. Carla was experiencing high-altitude insomnia. She hadn't slept more than a few hours each night. It was starting to wear on her, but she was determined to press on. As was I.

The trek to Mawenzi Tarn Camp would take three to four hours. It was a short but steep hike-no more than ones I had done in the past, but the altitude was starting to make the trek more challenging.

As we made our final approach to the camp, I started to feel wobbly. I couldn't quite get my hiking poles in the right place. Lasti grabbed my arm as we were scrambling over large boulder—like rock formations.

"*Pole, pole*, Mama Kubwa," he reminded me.

I know, I know, I thought. I started to get a headache. I drank gulp after gulp of water. I didn't feel better. I popped some Tylenol. Still the headache ground away at my skull.

Soon, my "perky, let's go" attitude turned into a sour, saucy one.

I didn't want help even though I needed it. I was whiny about everything. I didn't notice a beautiful pool of water or the shadow of Mawenzi peak towering above. I could barely look up.

I decided to soldier on-and join my group in the mess tent.

Popcorn, which had been so comforting alongside a white plastic mug filled with reddish Kenyan tea, milk powder and sugar, slithered in my teeth as I grew weary of gnawing. Popcorn was our trail's end snack that we shared in the green glow of the mess tent.

In the first few days of the journey, the mess tent was a portal for soul sharing, as laughter echoed in our nearly vacant Rongai Route campgrounds. On this day, though, the laughter was piercing. I didn't tell anyone about my headache because I didn't want to call attention to my misery.

I tugged my sweater over my wrists, and locked my thumb in the hole at the end of each sleeve, which I later used to wipe my nose. I clasped the cup with both hands and finished my tea, which had turned cold minutes after I had poured it. Excess sugar and milk powder had gathered together in a sticky lump on the cup's bottom.

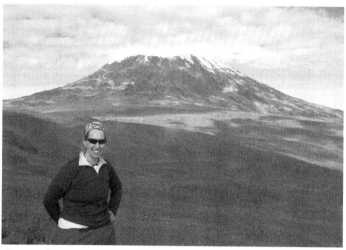

Getting closer. Two more days of hiking remained before I reached the top of Mount Kilimanjaro.

I needed to stop and take a break. So I headed to my tent.

I bowed out of the afternoon's acclimatization hike up a knife-edge ridge, even though I worried it would hamper my chances of getting up the mountain. I needed to take care of myself in this moment. I pulled myself into my sleeping bag, which Chris—who was feeling back up to speed—had set up for me.

I remember our itinerary had said, "You may well be starting to feel the effects of the altitude. It is not impossible for acute mountain sickness to occur even at this attitude, in which case your climb-leader will call for an immediate evacuation down the mountain. Under these circumstances, do not let any other thought of the summit cross your mind, but just get down the mountain as reasonably and safely as possible."

I lifted my arm over my eyes hoping this wouldn't be the summit of the mountain for me.

I didn't want my journey to end here. It astounded me that I was able to push on all this way after having been stuck in obesity for more than a decade. Perhaps I realized that my weight was a life and death situation. If I didn't start heading down a healthy path all could be lost in the way of diabetes, heart disease and more. I needed to keep moving in the right direction. I rolled over and did my best to take in deep breaths and calm myself into sleep.

13. DESERT DAYDREAM

By morning time, I had recovered. Sleeping and letting my body adjust to the altitude seemed to work. I needed to trust my body to do what was best for me. I felt groggy, but pressed on.

We had spent days winding our way up Kilimanjaro. Its square top loomed in the distance, growing ever closer. As we cleared a ridge after leaving Mawenzi Tarn Camp, we headed directly toward it. This was the final stretch before the steep summit attempt.

It looked like an easy segment of the trail, but it was far from it. The four or five hours across the saddle—between the two volcanoes of Mawenzi and the towering Kibo peak of Kilimanjaro—would be the hardest flat hike I had ever done.

It was indeed the plateau. All we could do was keep our heads down and keep moving forward. By this point in the trek, the laughter that kept us smiling during hikes was mostly gone. Conversation lulled into grunts, and whines were the way we spoke. Most of us didn't say anything at all. We just wanted to get there already as the mountain loomed ahead. *Come on, come on.*

We would hike for an hour and stop to drink water. It felt like we had barely covered any distance. It was like being on a

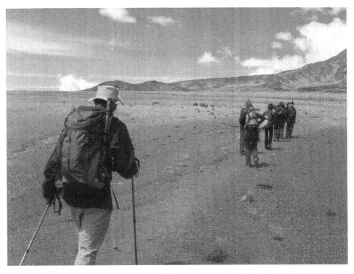

A stop along the alpine desert section of the mountain—the hardest flat hike of my life. We had to stop every hour to rest. Many of us were miserable, such as Lisa (bottom right) who tried to recover from her headache.

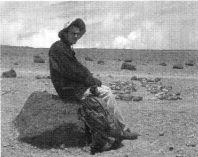

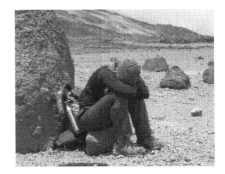

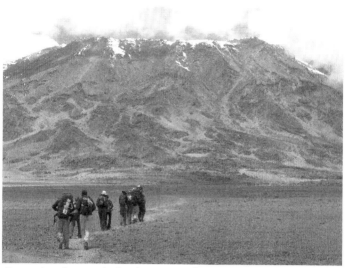

Onward and upward. Our base camp for the summit attempt was still hours away.

slow treadmill in the middle of nowhere.

There is a feeling of being at center stage, below Kilimanjaro's summit, which still, even four days in, seemed taller than any mountain I had hiked. We were still tiny little dots compared to the big square top of Kilimanjaro ahead.

We stopped at some big boulders in the middle of this vast stretch of nothingness and plunked ourselves down. There was something so strange and exposed about being on the way to Kibo Hut.

I asked Meke if he could point to where we were going. He pointed to a hut. Before this, we had been rather isolated from hikers—on our own path. We were about to merge with the Marangu route, a more traveled path up the mountain.

I could see little dots of hikers making their way up the mountain in colorful parkas and stopping at the base of the crest. At this pace, it felt like we would never get there. But eventually, step after step, we did. Our crew of porters had already set up our tents. All we wanted to do was lay down, but we had to eat a quick dinner before bed.

This was the night before summit night—twelve to fifteen hours of hiking, which was to begin at midnight.

For most of the porters, this was the end of the road. From here, we were to go with our guides up the remaining portion of the mountain, so there was a feeling of celebration in the air as we tried to sleep. Maybe it was mountain insomnia. Maybe it was nerves. But I didn't remember getting much sleep at all.

As I sat in my tent, restless, I heard the music from my yoga class. It must have been right around the time that my class was being held. My fellow yogis had promised to send me thoughts of strength—and it was coming through.

I thought about all the people who helped me up the mountain. I thought about all the orphans I was helping. I hoped I would make it to the top for all of them.

14. STEP. BREATHE.
STEP. BREATHE.

M y body was already fighting to stay alive in the oxygen-depleted environment. Even though I was completely still, my heart beat as if I were on the elliptical trainer. It was the sound of an easier workout, but nonetheless, I could hear my heart working.

Thump. Thump.

Thump. Thump.

Thump. Thump.

I was glad to have made it through the night. Knowing how little oxygen there was to go around, I feared when we were sent to bed at about 7 p.m. that I wouldn't take big enough gulps of air, suffocating in my sleep.

I think I woke up at about 10:30 p.m. I didn't look at the clock, fearing I'd jostle it too much (if I accidentally turned it off, I was sure I'd fall back asleep and miss the whole thing), or click on my headlamp and awaken Chris. These hours of sleep before the summit attempt were precious.

After all, summit day amounted to fifteen hours of hiking (not including breaks).

I quietly started to slip on the layers needed for this long-awaited leg of the journey. It started with long underwear, top and bottom. I took off my sleeping socks and put on sock liners, a thin cream-colored layer to prevent blisters, followed by heavy-weight hiking socks. I reached my arms up toward the top of the tent to put on my Icebreaker wool sweater, then a red fleece, a Christmas gift from my mother, and then a thick black one. Once my top layers were tucked in, I pulled on my snow pants, one leg at a time, looped the suspenders over my shoulders, and zipped the zipper to make sure they still fit.

I made sure my hat, mittens and neck gaiter (a fuzzy fleece to close the gap between my neck and nose) were in view. I put them at the end of my tent, next to my jacket and boots, which had hand warmers inside but were cold by the time I put them on and laced them up.

Exhausted from dressing, I laid back down on my sleeping bag. As I slumped back, I felt myself slide slightly down the mountain's pitch when the length of my Gore-Tex snow pants met the nylon exterior of my sleeping bag.

I heard steps and then the sound of a long plastic zipper going up. It was our wakeup call.

"Good morning," Robbie said, as he poked his head into our tent.

It was 11:30 p.m. If it weren't for Robbie's headlamp, I wouldn't have been able to see him through the thick, piercing darkness.

When Chris woke up, he was somewhat surprised to see me already in gear.

The trick of a successful summit attempt is to tackle the hardest parts of a climb first, while the winds are low and the sun is down. Since the hardest part on Kilimanjaro (up to Gilman's Point) takes seven hours, followed by a three-hour loop to Uhuru Peak and back, the summit attempt starts at midnight. But the summit isn't the end of it, because what goes up must come down.

In other words, there was no time to dawdle, which is troublesome since an oxygen-starved body starts to fumble. It took Chris a half hour to put his gaiters on the right way. He had never tested them and started with them backwards, trying to squeeze them over his boots. Robbie had to help him.

Chris and I made our way to the mess tent. I was roasting already. It was 24 degrees, downright balmy for summit night. Guides said it can be as cold as minus 25 degrees on the mountain top. I shivered just thinking about that.

I had one less layer than Meke suggested the previous evening. I skipped the clunky, fake North Face jacket.

Lauren and I both felt bulky and overheated. We contemplated shaving off a piece of clothing before we started. We were reminded that it would get colder as the climb went up and the night went on.

"The weather is unpredictable," Meke said, as he did every time we asked about what the conditions would be like the following day. Still, in our Weather Channel-crazed minds, we'd hang on to the end of the sentence, hoping there would be some kind of report about what to expect.

Ann wore a digital thermometer around her neck, but that only told us what it was at the moment. Meke was right. There is no way of knowing what storm would blow in when. It had rained for a week straight before our arrival. The day before our climb began, it snowed on the peak. So far, the weather was mild and mellow, and we were grateful. Rain can make for a miserable climb and turn the mountain into an ice-slicked slope. What would it matter anyway? It was our day to summit.

Chris looked groggy and unsettled across the table. I bet I did, too. We all did. (Yes, even Shawna. She wore black, thick-rimmed glasses and grasped her stomach as she ugh-ed through the forced meal.)

Then, Carla walked in the mess tent.

In the five days of walking together, we kept track of each others' ailments. We knew who couldn't poop. We knew who had diarrhea. Carla was the one we worried about the most. In addition to feeling a constant tinge of intestinal upset, she couldn't sleep. It wasn't the kind of insomnia that that kept her awake an hour or two longer than the rest of us. Insomnia is perhaps the cruelest high-altitude ailment: even after hours of exhausting hiking, some people can't sleep. Carla was hit hard. No matter how much she tried, whatever time she settled down, she couldn't relax. In four nights, her total sleep amounted to an hour, maybe two. When she walked in the tent, we looked at her, hoping that she had finally rested.

"I'm not going to lie. I didn't," Carla said without being asked. Her skin was ghostly white and her eyes were sunken and lost. I was amazed that instead of curling up and going back to bed, she suited up for the final stretch of the mountain.

The breakfast table, normally a celebratory start to our daily hikes, was stark with oatmeal in one pot (which most people passed on) and a dull silver platter of stale biscuits. Our chef, Trophine, set out only bland foods, which people can best stomach at 15,000 feet and higher.

I served myself a bowl of oatmeal. It was instantly cold but I ate it. Chris did, too. We had to. We were burning calories at an astronomical rate, just sitting there. This was eating for energy, I thought.

Trophine sent us on our way with two packs of biscuits and two bars of chocolate-double our normal dose. The palm-sized Cadbury chocolate bars were an exciting treat at the start of the journey. (They give us chocolate?) By now I had come to realize they were just warped little rectangles coated in a light brown powder, a sign they were past their prime. I had no real interest in the confection.

We all had Clif bars and trail snacks in our bags to eat the whole way up the mountain, though Lauren and I seemed to be the only ones with an appetite.

Nausea never bothered me. Even during some of my worst college drinking episodes I could stomach the alcohol. While my friends heaved, arms wrapped around a porcelain toilet, I'd hold their hair back.

It was as if I trained my stomach by stretching it, suffering through the likes of entire packages of Double Stuffed Oreos. I couldn't stop eating until the package was empty. I'd lick my fingers and press them into the black crumbs, trying scoop up every one I could. So, no, I never felt nauseous on Kilimanjaro.

I finished breakfast and tactfully dropped brown iodine tablets and pink grapefruit-flavored Airborne tablets in our Camelbaks. It was impossible to boil drinking water at this altitude. This batch had been dredged from a stagnant lake and carried to the Kibo campsite. I wanted safe drinking water to be the least of my worries, because I had plenty of other ones about the journey ahead.

It was about 12:30 a.m., time to hit the trail. I clicked on my headlamp and stepped out of the mess tent.

"*Twende. Twende*," Meke said. The Swahili words for "Let's go. Let's go," used to make me smile, as I shared Meke's enthusiasm to get up the mountain. Now that we were on our summit attempt, they scared me.

I tried to slide the Camelbak in my backpack, but it wiggled like a live fish. I hurried and dropped it. I spewed several profanities, dusted it off, and got in line. I was number three, behind Lauren and Carla. I remembered when Carla told the group during dinner of day two, "I thought I should let you know, I'm a fainter. It happens when I'm sick, like when I have a fever." And perhaps, when she hasn't slept? I admired Carla, but at the same time worried that she was going to hurt herself, or others. I worried she'd fall back on me.

I asked, "Are you sure you're okay?"

She didn't answer. I had no idea what to expect on this leg of the journey. As we settled into our tents the previous evening, the summit and our campground were encased in clouds. A few flakes of snow drifted down as we rested our heads. The slope was hard to gauge. The trails weren't marked; there was no railing, not even a distinct path that one could see in the daylight. Now that it was dark, we could see nothing but the few feet in front of us where our headlamps shone. All I could see in front of me was the back of Carla's head.

Marching in the dark takes faith. Each step was in line with our leader, hoping the rhythm of his footsteps would take us in the right direction. I didn't have any idea where I was going. I figured as long as we were going up, we were okay.

We cleared the campground, through the blackest darkness I'd ever experienced, and saw a few other bands of headlamps higher up on the mountainside. They looked like stars wriggling toward the summit. As we walked up and up, the real stars encircled us.

I wanted to grasp the enormity of it all. I started to tense up because this was it—the summit day. Even the itinerary promoting our trip called it "a nightmare."

The scree surface, like clumps of kitty litter, was treacherous and unstable. Sometimes it took three steps, with feet sliding back, to travel one step's pace. I had read about scree in guidebooks. I thought about practicing by walking up piles of gravel in quarries but never did, for fear of being swallowed by the pile of chipped rock.

I tried to remember anything from Kilimanjaro climb guidebooks about what to expect. But then again, it didn't matter. The landscape was invisible. When I looked down, I could see my feet, moving one slow step at a time. When I looked back, I could see headlamps bobbing in unison. When I let my headlamp shine down the path I had just traveled, it sloped so steeply downward that it scared me. The quiet panic that started to set in my mind was interrupted by the sound of Lasti's voice.

He started singing what he later told me were Swahili love songs and lullabies. Robbie and James joined in. They cooed for hours, singing when we fought to breathe. Their words washed over us, carried us:

> *Nami nisemeje*
> *Kijana mwenzio*
> *Nashindwa na mali sina wee*
> *Ningekuoa malaika*
> *Malaika nakupenda malaika*

Nobody talked. We walked and listened. We listened to the songs. We listened to the sound of our exaggerated breath.

Step. Breathe. Step. Breathe.

It was a one-Mississippi, two-Mississippi pace. Even then, about an hour into the nighttime journey, people fell back. Carla moved toward the back of the line. I moved to the front, with Lauren or Chris behind me.

"I could really go for Taco Bell right now. Something warm, cheesy. A burrito, maybe," Lauren said.

Her words kind of surprised me. For once, I hadn't been thinking about food. Breathing and walking was enough. Though the only thing I'd consider leaving the mountain for, after days of peeing behind rocks and pooping in a common pot, would be a gorgeous, porcelain toilet. Lauren was with me on that one. On night three, she dreamt that she missed summit day because she went on a bus to visit a beautiful bathroom.

Meke stopped and said to me, "It helps the others to let them catch up."

Each word became encircled by a cloud, lit by my headlamp. I was glad, glad to have any break. Sometimes he would go on and I'd think about asking for a break, but hoped someone else would ask for one first.

I stopped and let my headlamp shine down the mountain. I felt a twinge of vertigo; I decided that I would only look forward.

Lasti, Robbie, and James would walk up the line, asking each person how they were. They looked at us for a moment to make sure we weren't lying.

James would say, "Mama Kubwa, are you okay?"

"Great," I said, running out of breath by the "T."

"Full, deep-belly breathing," I said to myself and then to Chris, who was behind me. In my Zen mindset, I repeated reminders from my yoga instructor, "Where's the breath?"

"Worry about yourself," Chris said, as he turned to find a place to sit. I knew that look, that annoyed look. Perhaps it was because I reminded him how to breathe at every break.

Meke turned to me and said, "When we're resting, we should be drinking. Not talking."

I shut up and drank. A few minutes later, we started again.

Meke called down the mountain to people behind us. "Don't give up the fight. This is how we do it. We just walk, walk, and walk."

We walked, walked, and walked.

Walking and breathing was my meditation. Step. Breathe. Step. Breathe. Nothing else mattered. The higher we climbed, the harder it was.

Two hours into the night's trail, I was still in the lead. In the months before the climb I had worried that I would be last in line. The kind of last in line like I was on middle school field trips, holding up the bus while everyone waited for me to return, red-faced and sweaty. Now I was first, even ahead of Chris, who started to feel sick while chomping through a frozen Power Bar.

"Williams Point," Meke announced. "We're now higher than Mawenzi Peak."

I remembered the towering, jagged peak of Mawenzi above the campground on our third night. My brain was in a headache vice and I hoped dexamethasone, my altitude sickness medication, would work. I wondered, looking up at Mawenzi, Kilimanjaro's sister peak, if I would be able to go on. Mawenzi seemed so high, so impossible and yet thousands of feet shorter than Kilimanjaro. Now I was past it.

I breathed in heavy through my nose and grinned as my headlamp illuminated the sign.

"Williams Point: 5,000 m."

That's 16,404 feet above sea level. Uhuru Peak was just 2,939 feet away-the hardest 2,939 feet of the climb.

FAT WOMAN ON THE MOUNTAIN

15. DARKEST BEFORE DAWN

We kept on and on through the night until Hans Meyer Cave. Hans Meyer is the guy who first climbed Kilimanjaro—at least, the first documented person. It was before World War I and lots of curious Europeans visiting Africa wanted to know could there really be snow 200 miles from the Equator. Plus, back then, Europeans loved conquering things. By then much of Africa was colonized by one European country or another.

Plenty of people tried to climb Kilimanjaro but failed. In 1861, German explorer Baron Von der Decken and English geologist R. Thornton tried to get to Kilimanjaro's summit, but bad weather cut their climb short below the forest line. Der Decken returned the following year with Dr. Otto Kersten. They climbed in heavy snow and reached 14,107 feet, the elevation where we slept on our third night of the mountain. An Austro-Hungarian team of Count Samuel Teleke and Lt. Ludwig von Holnel also tried, but got to 15,797 feet, just above where Kibo Camp now stands, before turning back.

Meyer, a German geologist, decided to give it a go in 1887. It would take him three attempts to get to the top of the mountain. He finally reached in 1889.

Lots of the things were named after Meyer on and near the

mountain. (By the way, the first woman who climbed to Gilman's Point was Frau von Ruckteschell, but I didn't see anything named after her.) Out of all the things named after Meyer, I remembered Hans Meyer Cave the most.

During our pre-climb not-so-pep talk, our trip coordinator told us if someone were going to give up, turn back, it would likely happen at Hans Meyer Cave. The cave can be a physical, emotional, or mental breaking point for many climbers. It's the point, after three hours of hiking, when wandering out in the dark isn't as new and exciting as it was about midnight under a canopy of stars.

A meditation of step, breath, and the songs from our porters had carried us up the first few hours of the mountain. But now it was just dull and dark. And hard. Breath was hard to come by, sometimes taking as much energy as it did to step. This was the time when the mind starts to wander. *Is this ever going to end?*

The pace had grown tiresome, with the constant grind of gravel under boot, knowing the day's climb is not even halfway through. Not even a third. It was colder the higher we got. It had dropped five degrees to 19.

I had to forget what the trip coordinator said and think positively. I had to remember that the summit was close to Hans Meyer Cave (16,896 feet)—maybe just a couple of hours more until the ridge, Gilman's Point (18,652 feet). *You can do anything for a couple of hours. It's just a couple of hours of your life.*

I tried to visualize the hand-drawn map tucked in my backpack, trying to pinpoint Hans Meyer Cave on the mountain's slope. I figured it was about halfway between where we started that night and Gilman's Point. It must have been about 4 a.m.

So, even when it came time to take a break at Hans Meyer

Cave, I convinced myself that I was still revving, charging to go. Besides, I couldn't even see this so-called Hans Meyer Cave in the dark. I would not give up, not now.

I was the only one in my group who didn't find a rock to sit down on. I opted against it after my headlamp shined on the remnants of other people taking a pit stop there—toilet paper strewn on the rocks and ground, and hardened excrement between the rocks. I decided to stand.

After I stopped, I heard the other climbers coming up behind me in the dark, the sound of feet dragging on a gravel driveway. One by one, they found a spot to sit and rest. My headlamp shined on the face of each climber who reached the resting spot. Their eyes looked tired. Their breathing was heavy.

Our leader Ann, who many said could walk to the summit in high heel shoes, and Lauren, the high-altitude living ski bum, were the only perky ones.

My cheerleader, Sarah, and my idol, Shawna, were dragging. The world spun beneath their feet. Sarah felt dizzy but didn't want to eat. She hadn't eaten much if anything at breakfast hours earlier. Robbie gave her a glucose gel packet, the kind of carbohydrate punch that cyclists pound while on the road. It dripped down her throat, and eventually made her feel better.

Chris, whose stomach swirled with nausea, had plunked himself on a rock away from the others. Still, he knew we needed to eat. He offered me a piece of a Power Bar. Frozen, it felt like a brick on my front teeth. I tried to wash it down with water. I bit down on my Camelbak mouthpiece and tried to pull water through the tube. Some water came, but not much. The pencil-thin tube connection between my mouth and the bag of water hanging in my backpack was starting to freeze (even with the thermal sleeve that I paid $25 for to cover it). My cocktail of vitamins and water purification tablets tasted like a pink grapefruit and iodine Slurpee.

Lisa had fallen behind. When she got to Hans Meyer Cave, she slumped down and immediately checked in with tent-mate Lauren, making sure she had enough Diamox. Lauren and Lisa had never met before the climb, but from the moment they started walking together up the mountain, they watched over each other in the way that sisters would.

The crowd was mostly quiet, silently grateful for the rest, or mumbling about how tired we were. Then, Carla announced in the dark, "This is way harder than a marathon." My headlamp shined on her face, a spotlight as she spoke slumped down on the rock. "A marathon is four hours, and when you're finished all of your friends bring you food. Here, we have to hike for four days, and even when we're done, we have to walk miles for our dinner."

I heard a few muffled chuckles around me in the dark. We had to get to the summit before we could even think about dinner. I spun my headlamp around to survey who was there and how they looked. Where was Karen?

Karen showed up just as we were about to start going again. Robbie told the group to go on, and they would catch up later. They never would. Karen later described her high-altitude headache, which began three days prior, like a vice that crunched her head, and turned tighter with each step. At Hans Meyer Cave, it became unbearable. She had to go arm and arm with Robbie down the mountain.

Typically the best and only cure for altitude sickness symptoms is to go down the mountain. Every extra sip of oxygen helps heal the ailing body. Even knowing that before getting on the mountain doesn't make it an easy decision once

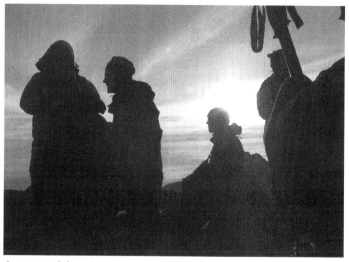

Sunrise at Gilman's Point.

we were there. It's easy to succumb to summit fever, an obsessive desire to get to the top of the mountain. Some ailing climbers demand to be carried the rest of the way.

Karen was about three hours from Gilman's Point, where she would have earned a green certificate from the Tanzanian Park Service for her efforts, four and a half hours to the real summit, Uhuru. For that she would have earned a gold certificate, and huddled in for a photo at the summit sign.

But Karen had been a nurse and she knew better than to continue on. She knew her body was telling her not to. Deciding to turn back may have taken more strength than the actual climb.

By the next rest stop, word traveled up the line of climbers that Karen had gone down the mountain for her own safety. It was heartbreaking for her. It was heartbreaking for all of us.

Not everyone who tries to hike Kilimanjaro makes it to the

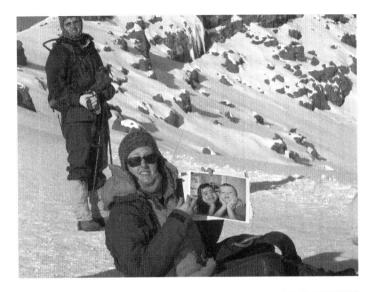

Above: Sarah and a photo of her daughters.

Right: Lauren anxious to get moving to the summit.

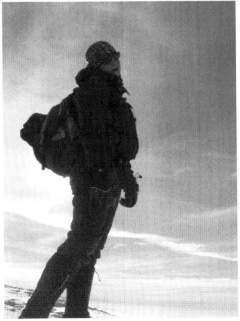

top. We knew someone would most likely have to retreat. The implication was in every question about the odds of who makes it up the mountain. The odds were that two people in our group wouldn't make it up Kilimanjaro. I hoped the second wouldn't be me. There were still hours to go with the reality of someone else exiting our journey haunting my steps.

We were back moving up the mountain, onto the next section called the zigzags, the doldrums of the trail. That blind faith that carried me through the first few hours behind Meke had dissolved.

Unlike the long, graceful, wide switchback trails carved into of the Grand Canyon, Meke weaved back and forth, wobbling and weaving like a drunken snake. The scree was especially granular here, slipping under our footfalls a lot more frequently as the early morning continued.

I felt like we were going nowhere. I was used to being led. When it comes to travel or hiking, Chris is the navigator, I am the communicator. I'm used to the fact that Chris is a bit of a map hog when it came to hiking, but there always comes a time in each journey that I demand to see our trail on paper.

I tried to watch the trail under Meke's feet and to see its direction further up the mountain, but my headlamp would only light so far ahead of us. I worried he was lost and making his steps up as we went along. The singing was a little more sporadic now. The group was silent, aside from sniffles and the grunts and groans of exhaustion.

"People forget this part," Meke said. I had heard climbing Kilimanjaro is a lot like childbirth. After you experience the exuberance of reaching the summit, you forget how hard it was to get there. If that's the case, summit night is like labor. "They forget it's hard. That it takes so long," Meke confided in me. He must have thought since I was still one or two people behind him that I was strong enough to handle such commentary. But I, too, was pushing.

I had to sit. I should have done it back at Hans Meyer Cave. I was sure someone else would ask for a break. So I waited.

Breathe. Breathe. Step. Breathe. Breathe. Step.

Bathroom breaks aside, I had never been the one to ask for a rest break from hiking in our five days together. There were typically plenty of breaks built in along the route, or someone else just wanted to rest. I didn't want to be the one to ask. I didn't want people to think that I was giving up, that I was too exhausted to go on.

I hadn't been the one who asked until that moment, about thirty minutes from our last break. Five hours into the slowest pace I'd ever walked, I said it. "Stop, I need to stop."

Meke found a nondescript spot where we plunked our butts on the dusty, rocky ground, the terrain we had spent the last hour sloughing over.

By now, water wasn't coming out of my tube, not at all. The Camelbak tube was a rigid popsicle under the plastic. I needed to grab my water bottle from my backpack.

It was hard handling things with the clunky gloves that were thick enough to keep me warm in the now 17-degree cold. I took them off, and pawed through my backpack using a thin black pair of liners that gave little more coverage than a pair of women's white tea gloves. I fumbled around the straps and buckles of my backpack to grasp my bottle of water which had also frozen partially, sparking in the light of my headlamp. I drank a bit, offered some to Chris. I let out an "Ah" as I drank, sat, and relaxed. My breath formed a cloud in front of my mouth. Naptime, I thought.

I kept the big clunky gloves off. My fingers felt free, but they were freezing by the second. I didn't have the energy to put the gloves back on.

When Meke said we had two more minutes before continuing, I sat still. I didn't bother to suit up again. I hadn't rested long enough the last time, so I figured I better soak in as much as I could.

After most of my fellow climbers suited up and stood, I tried to get up as well but felt like my hands didn't work. My fingertips were frozen, tingly. It could have been the beginning of frostbite, just like I had felt in Telluride when I decided to turn back during a day of training. I felt like needles were piercing through my nails. I tried to shake my hands and squeeze them together. But it didn't help.

When Lauren had chilly fingers a few minutes before, Robbie took out a hand warmer and held them tight on her hands. He rubbed them and she smiled. I wanted the same treatment. Now that I was complaining of the same, if not worse ailment, everyone stood mute, seemingly annoyed that I was delaying the trip up the mountain. I knew I had hand warmers, even foot warmers, in my backpack, but I couldn't get to them.

"Does anyone have spare hand warmers in an accessible spot?" I asked. I just felt the headlamps looking back at me. "Mine are deep in my backpack. I can't get my hands to work."

I wanted to cry when no one responded. I felt like the fat girl being left out again. I realized this is the part when the climb is an individual feat, not a group effort. Finally, I asked Ann directly, "Do you have any?"

She took some out of her bag and handed them to me. It hurt me to curl my fingers around them. Finally, I started to get mobility in them, just not much. Meke decided it was time to get going again.

"Not much longer until Jamaica Rocks," he told me. "Twende, twende."

I wanted to get back behind him. Maybe even behind Lauren, but with the time it took to thread my hands through the loops of my hiking poles I joined the line four or five climbers behind him. Right behind Chris.

I was sure my fingertips were frostbitten. My head was starting to feel woozy. It was dark but I knew Gilman's Point, where many call an end to their climb, was still two hours away. I had seen headlamps disappear over the ridge. I wondered if I would make it there.

I was annoyed that I wasn't in front any longer. I liked being there. Anytime I tried to rush myself, I would get winded, spent. I bumbled my way up as my legs started to get that lead-like weight, my feet dragged deeper in the scree.

"Ugh," I would grunt, taking in a deep breath, and tilt my head up to the heavens between steps. I think I was praying. Another hour. Please give me another hour of strength. I'd sink my poles into the ground, and take a deep exaggerated breath in before taking the next step forward. And then again. And again. And again.

It was hard to be lost in the movement, moving was so hard. My brain was engaged in a battle between telling myself I couldn't do it and the conviction that I spent so long focusing on: that I'd make it to the summit.

Each step was a struggle.

My headlamp shined ahead, and lit the immediate landscape—which looked like a Maine beach strewn with rocks, but vertical. We had arrived at Jamaica Rocks—5,500 meters.

I wanted to be excited. We had reached the third major

landmark on our quest to get to Gilman's Point and beyond. I wanted a nap. We all wanted a nap. This was where I'd have to start scrambling over boulders, using balance, strength, and courage to make it up the rest of the mountain. I wondered if I had any left.

We rested again at the base of Jamaica Rocks. The terrain, while at times dusted with the scree-like surface on its engraved trails, reminded me of Bear Mountain in upstate New York. I had taken my new sturdy-enough-for-Kilimanjaro boots there for a test drive. It was where I learned to trust my feet.

It had been hard to part with my old canvas boots, since they had been with me for so much of my journey, including the Grand Canyon. I wore them even though they nearly rubbed the knuckle off my second toe each time I descended down a mountain. For Kilimanjaro, I needed a pair of sturdy, leather boots.

When first I started hiking in my new boots just two months before the Kilimanjaro climb, it felt like ten-pound rocks were strapped to my feet. I found myself, wobbly, making excuses about not moving fast. These boots were heavy.

Suddenly, I realized that this is the way I felt when I was heavier and had just started hiking. I was focused on my weight instead of moving forward. Instead of thinking of my new boots as a burden, I started to think of them as my new tools. At first I wanted to crawl up the slant. Then I learned to trust my feet and myself, and eventually, I stood upright, and let my boots work for me, instead of me working against them.

I had agility, and even more power. My feet climbed over some boulders like a tank. When going downhill, I had so much more cushion. Instead of the jarring of my toes hitting the front of my boots like they did in my old faithful canvas pair, I felt secure with any step up or down the mountain. It reminded me of the importance of having a good mental state as you climb. If you think about falling you will. If you are looking for the next safe step, you will find it.

Perhaps I had been feeling so spent because my dose of dexamethasone was wearing off. It was 6 a.m. and time for another pill. I sent it down my dry throat with a swig of water.

I spent the break thinking about how I had climbed the hardest part, the scree field. I was now in familiar territory, rocks. Sure, I was a world away from Mount Tammany, Bear Mountain, and Camel's Hump, but when it came to the terrain of Jamaica Rocks, I had been there, done that. Jamaica Rocks were not any more challenging. Now the challenge was keeping my mind and body in a positive state.

I realized I didn't have to lead anymore. I did that enough for one night. I needed to go at my pace. "*Pole, pole.*" Because this is where it counted, the last hour in the dark to feel focused and strong.

"Don't give up the fight," Meke called down the line. "*Twende.*"

That's right, I thought, *Twende. Give it all you've got.*

It wasn't easy. At times my limbs felt heavy and constricted, under layers of padding. Other times they were limp like a ragdoll's, overshooting the spot where I wanted to step.

Lasti told me it was best to abandon my poles. My hiking poles had been my safety net, helping me power through strides, but now I was on my own. I grabbed onto rocks where I felt I would get the most leverage to lift myself to the next step.

"Take your time," he'd say to me, or to anyone rushing themselves.

There was no rush. Each step was all I had at that moment.

It was all I had to do.

My mind looked at the rock formations ahead of me. I'd scope out the hobbled grooves, finding the next spot to go. After two deep breaths, I'd launch one foot up. It was important to get it right, to focus. The wrong step could mean a twisted ankle or slipping off the surface and tumbling down for who knows how long.

It was steep here, and slow. I lost track of time. It was cold and I didn't dare ask anyone to expose their wrists to look at their watches. Who wants to be the "Are we there yet" kid? I knew we were, indeed, nearly there. I tried to remember that. My eyes were fixed on my feet, making their way up the mountain, one tiring pace at a time.

The puzzle of the rock formations was a distraction. I kept looking down, using the light of my headlamp to point me in the right direction. I'd watch the steps of the people in front of me, especially Chris, and follow their lead. Sometimes, I'd see another way, an easier way along the rocks, and I'd smile and nod to myself. "Good girl."

I hadn't even noticed that the light from my headlamp wasn't the only light showing the path.

"Here it is, the sunrise," someone called.

I turned my sleepy head to the right to see a soft orange glow in the sky. We let out a collective, "Whoa." Within minutes, the sun's rays shot out behind Mawenzi's jagged peak. We were so much higher than Mawenzi. We dwarfed it. We couldn't see our campsite below. We were in a totally different realm.

As we watched, dumbfounded by the sunrise's beauty, it was as though we each collected the solar energy, refilling our reserves. It was the most animated I had seen the group in more than a day. We all smiled.

The sun lit the path in front of us. Gilman's Point was no more than two flights of stairs away. We could see we would make it if we just kept walking.

While the others continued to walk up, I leaned against the rocks and pulled out my video camera to capture the sunrise. Soon everyone had gone ahead, the final push to the first peak. Everybody but Lasti.

He asked, "Are you okay? Are you dizzy?"

"I'm great. I'm great. This is just so beautiful."

16. DAY 5: FREEDOM. UHURU PEAK

Taking time to videotape the sunrise made me last in line. I could see my climbing companions' hats just over the ridge of the rock.

I was so excited to be there, one flight away from Gilman's Point, that I started to rush to be part of the celebration of making it this far. I walked without breathing and started to wobble on the last jagged rock steps.

"Are you dizzy? *Pole, pole*," Lasti commanded and grabbed my hiking sticks so I could regain my balance on the rocks.

He was right. I needed to slow down. No matter how slow I went, it wouldn't take long to get to Gilman's Point. I was a mere ten steps away. Those ten steps took about ten minutes to negotiate and conquer, harnessing my hands around the volcanic rock, securing my next step and vaulting myself upward. But I was so excited.

Chris, who had been videotaping my final steps up, embraced me, our jackets making that swishy nylon sound against each other. The celebration was short since I, like others in the group, became fascinated by the view at Gilman's Point, which was like a tree house where you could survey the world below. We were so high that the horizon below was curved, offering a glimpse of the rocky Kilimanjaro region and the surrounding plains. The path I had finished looked straight down-dropping off in the distance. The sky above was already a brilliant blue, while the horizon was a pink striation of clouds.

Once safely within Gilman's Point, it looked like a giant robin's nest of rock, littered with the wrappers of celebratory Clif Bar and water bottles from other groups. The destination, marked by a standard brown and yellow park service sign announcing Gilman's Point, 5,686 meters above sea level, was a crowded place for climbers. Some wore rock-climbing helmets. I wondered, but didn't have the energy to ask, how they arrived there.

James handed me a cup of tea, signaling that it was finally morning. "Drink this," he said, as I tried to hold the white plastic cup in my thick black gloves. I took a seat toward the back of the Gilman's Point perch to watch the jubilant silhouettes against the horizon.

The Russian man who was next to me didn't look well. His guide looked worried. After months of reading about mountain climbing, the only thing that came to mind was to ask, "Ah, Russia. Have you done Elbrus?"

He gave me an "Are-you-kidding-me?" look, as if he never wanted to be on another mountain in his life, and didn't answer.

Many tours call Gilman's Point the summit, enough to earn a green certificate from the Tanzanian park service and turn back. For others, possibly including this Russian guy, turning back at Gilman's Point isn't a choice.

The true summit, Uhuru Peak, was another 1,000 feet away. I did the math months in advance, calculating the distance between Gilman's Point and Uhuru, so when it came time to make the choice between settling for a green certificate at Gilman's or going for the gold certificate I would earn at Uhuru,

I would go for the gold. I knew it was no more than ninety minutes away. It was no more than a practice mountain hike.

That wasn't enough to convince Lisa, who had settled into her own minor mountain madness, to continue. She bickered with Meke about not wanting to press on.

"Who the hell cares whether it's this summit or the other?" she justified.

"It's flat from here," Meke told her. That wasn't exactly true, though as she looked at the trail from Gilman's Point onward, it looked almost downhill. She decided to continue with the group.

"Fine," Lisa said, gathering her stuff to press on.

I finished my tea and tried to get my CamelBak to work. I flexed the long tube back and forth. Trying to encourage the water to warm under the ever-brightening sky was exhausting. Still nothing came out. I hadn't had a full drink of water for more than an hour even though my backpack was heavy from the weight of liquid still in my CamelBak.

The entire stop at Gilman's Point couldn't have been longer than fifteen minutes, so by the time I arrived, five minutes remained. My legs felt heavy and tired. I tried to convince Meke to stay a few more minutes.

"I haven't even posed for a photo in front of the sign, Meke," I said, probably sounding like a whiny child. Meke ignored me and started walking, leading the group behind Gilman's Point, onward to Uhuru Peak.

Meke was right to press forward as we had reached the point where the air held half as much oxygen as at sea level. He knew we couldn't last much longer up there. Breathing, even while only sitting down, was hard. The guides were now like cattle herders, making sure we were all well and on our way to the top so that we could make it back down again.

The good news was the sunlight brought new energy to the endeavor. There was a downright giddy feeling of having made it this far. The daylight, inviting me to fixate on the alien landscape ahead of us-plus the lightheaded euphoria of an oxygen-deprived mind-made it hard to focus.

The path of pure-white snow was dotted by the occasional rock jutting through. The snow creaked under boot, as if I were in some slow-motion mountaineering movie. I was making my own adventure flick. To be on top of this mountain—something that had been so imposing and such a life-long goal I had thought about all these months—felt as if I could accomplish anything step by step.

Nature was working for me. Suddenly, I realized that there was no wind to speak of. I had worried about Sarah's harrowing story of having to hold onto a guide her entire way up the mountain. For us, it was smooth sailing, and I was awash with gratitude.

The sun, perhaps magnified by my black jacket, black pants, and black hat, warmed my face. I finally could wear my sunglasses, which made it feel like the hike had finally begun.

The first leg of the journey was, to my relief, downhill. But that didn't mean it was easy. We treaded single file on the narrow path next to a rock wall. The ground was slick with ice and snow, and the guides knew to watch out for our tired legs. Lasti stayed with Chris and me. He made sure to point out each place to put my feet.

"Step here. And now here," he said, jumping down and in front of me, each part of the way. I was annoyed, because I was an experienced hiker. Now that I could see the path in front of me, I wanted to choose my steps. But I was too tired to make a fuss, and I had promised myself to trust the guides' judgment. I listened. I could have injured myself in a fall, and who knows what lay beneath the snow. Besides, I was in no mood to do more uphill climbing than I needed to. I didn't want any of the guides to be responsible for carrying me down the mountain.

Later, Lasti told me he was worried about me. He thought I might be getting sick from the altitude. I should have been onto it because he kept asking me how I was feeling. One wrong step could have sent me down a slope into what looked like a crater, though the true crater of Kilimanjaro's volcanic past was on the other side of the mountain.

Our pace was slow and fixed, so we arrived at Stella Point as a group. It felt just around the corner from Gilman's Point, because it was. With our oxygen-starved bodies, it took about forty-five minutes to get there.

It wasn't even 8 a.m. But being so high up, so close to the Equator, it was time to protect ourselves from the sun. I sat down on the snowy ground and shared a tube of 30-SPF sunscreen with Chris. It was icy-cold cream, having been attached to a carabineer clip on my backpack. I popped my sunglasses up onto my head and squinted my eyes-to protect them from sun blindness-as I covered the rest of my face with sun block.

Chris served up another half of an energy bar. I wasn't even hungry but I knew we needed to eat.

While the rest of the group sat, Lauren stood with the guides during the Stella Point stop. "Come on," she egged Meke on. Though we could see the last leg of our journey and other climbers making their way down, we needed a moment to gather strength.

"How was it?" I found myself calling out. They didn't stop to talk. They just kept moving down.

Sarah took out the photos of her two girls, readied it for the summit photos, while some of us suffered. Shawna clutched her head. Lisa was pissed; this was harder than just "a short summit walk." She wanted the climb to be over. It was time to go and get up off the ground. My butt was feeling icy anyway.

There is a balance to resting at high altitude. Rest too long and oxygen deprivation will get the best of you—from feeling faint to succumbing to the pure effort it takes to get to the top. On the other hand, not taking time to rest can slow the entire journey or stop it short. The body was not made to walk for twelve to fifteen hours straight, as we had set out to do on that Summit Day.

I felt like everything creaked when I bent one knee to launch myself up, off the cooling snow.

"Ugh," I said, using my hiking poles as leverage to lift the rest of myself up onto my feet.

From there, I got a great view of the glaciers. They looked like living, breathing beings, not just part of the horizon. They stand stoic in the distance with bluish vertical gills. James held my poles as I removed my glove from my now-warmed hand to take a photo of the massive ice shelves. I snapped a photo, thinking that if I climbed Kilimanjaro in another year or so, they might not be there. Sarah, who had been in the same spot two years prior, said the ice formations looked smaller and sick. I thought of Al Gore.

Then, I snapped a photo of James, who seemed in top form despite his duties on this journey. Instead of saying cheese, he bellowed out, "Mama Kubwa" and gave me an encouraging grin.

I looked at the path ahead, the last leg of our upward journey. On my normal training terrain, I would have thought of this last incline as little more than a hill. It looked so much like my Telluride training turf that I half expected someone to swish by me on a pair of skis. In fact, I stayed to the right of the trail, just in case.

"*Twende, twende*, Mama Kubwa," Meke said. In other words, get going.

I tried to temper myself, but couldn't help but charge ahead with the pack. Again, I was going too fast. I took a moment to press the weight of my body onto my poles and take a deep breath in through my nose. I felt little satisfaction. I did it twice more, to steady and calm my mind.

I was nearly there, but if I went too fast, too excitedly, I could lose it all. I didn't want to be carried down the terrain I had just conquered on my own two feet.

During my mini-break, the kind that seemed to happen every five paces or so, Lauren dropped her water bottle. It slipped down an incline and spun on a section of ice-slicked snow. Lasti quickly ran after it, making it down a ravine. I was amazed at his energy. He ran as quickly up the hill to rejoin the group, which included a doting Lauren. I realized the benefit of climbing up to the top of the mountain again and again, as was Lasti's job. He had spunk while the rest of us looked spent.

Watching the water bottle rescue cost me valuable time. Chris, who couldn't be bothered, continued on ahead, engrossed in his own footsteps.

I called out to him. "Baby, wait," I said. "Let's ... do this ... last part ... together."

He waited. I felt lead legged and frustrated that I couldn't run the five steps it would have taken to meet him. I closed my eyes and took a deep breath and another and another. Just one step at a time, and I would get there.

In my mind, I heard, "Thump. Thump. Thump."

It was the sound I heard while preparing for my trek in Colorado, the sound of Dennis' hands on his kitchen table. During my Telluride training, Dennis described what it takes to succeed during a high-altitude hike, or as he liked to call it, "mountain slogging."

"It's like this," Dennis said. He thumped one hand down on the table, waited an agonizing several seconds and did it again. My feet followed the rhythm of his tapping which played again and again in my mind like drums as Chris waited.

Suddenly my mind was flooded with images of everyone who had helped me on this journey—from those who cheered me on, to the more than 100 people who made donations on behalf of the climb. Their images and messages floated through my mind like a movie montage, set to the beat of Dennis' pace.

After about a dozen paces, I had arrived at Chris, my biggest and best supporter of all.

"Look where we are," he said. Up ahead, I could see clusters of people posing in front of a brown park sign, the one we had been moving towards for five days. I started to cry.

"You did it, sweetie. You did it," Chris said.

I wrapped my arms, still looped with hiking poles, around Chris and thanked him. Thanked him for being with me on this journey. I tried to wipe the tears from my face with my water-resistant glove. Instead, it smeared the salty liquid that quickly cooled my face, which was warm from the blazing sun. Tears continued to streak down my face as the climbing group before us cleared out and our Global Alliance for Africa group took our final steps to the top.

We handed our camera off to the guides and assembled as a group around the sign, trying not to hide the words: "Congratulations. You are now at Uhuru Peak, Tanzania, 5895

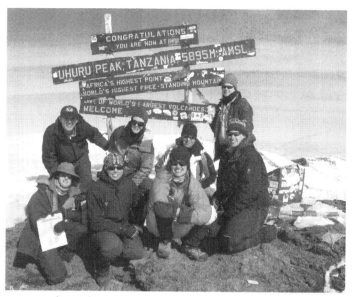

Front row from left to right: Chris, Anne, Lisa, Carla.
Bottom row: Sarah, Lauren, Shawna, Me.

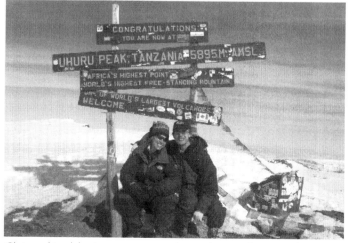

Chris and I celebrate a moment together at the top of Mount Kilimanjaro.

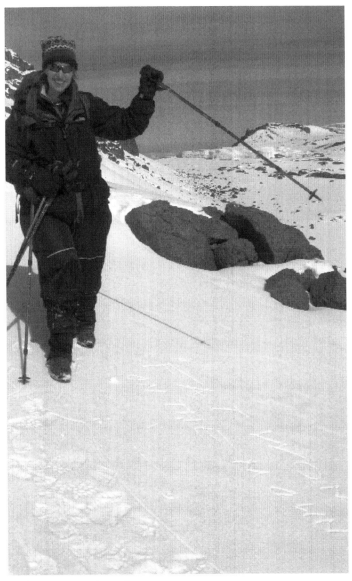

Making my way down the mountain.

M SMSL. Africa's highest point. World's Highest Freestanding Mountain. One of the World's Largest Volcanoes. Welcome."

The boards were dotted with stickers. Tibetan freedoms flags, with white, yellow, red and green banners, were slung on the posts.

My hamstrings were rope tight as I made my final steps. I needed to stretch. Instead of my normal sun salutation, a pose that I thought would eat up too much energy, I collapsed into child's pose, with my knees bent and my body spread forward over them, bowing in devotion to the mountain. I thanked my feet for being for being strong on the mountain and the m ountain for being strong under my feet. I was weepy as I realized that I had envisioned standing on top of this mountain for so long. Now, I was there. This mountain meant so much.

Uhuru is Swahili for "freedom," and I was there—free from a life that held me back, free to go anywhere I want.

17. SCREE RUNNING

Everyone started back, but I didn't feel like hurrying. I needed to. The 19,343-foot peak was not meant for living. Our hearts raced as we stood still. It was time to go down, Meke commanded.

Standing with the curved landscape around me, I tried to let it all sink in. It was too much. I conquered this goal-I made it up this mountain that I thought about going up for more than a year. I took a deep breath, and thought, *Wow. I am here, almost hypnotized by the scene.*

For once I didn't want to keep up. I wanted to bask in the celebratory atmosphere of the mountaintop, to know that I had done it.

I watched other climbers making their way up, and I wanted to embrace each one—as if to say, "Good job, I know how hard you've worked."

My internal play was interrupted by Meke, who had been standing, waiting with Lasti. "We need to get you down," he said. "*Twende.*"

With all of my visualization of going up the mountain, I never thought about going down. As everyone but Chris nearly trotted down the same slope that took us thirty minutes to traverse, I stayed put.

We watched as a few others used the wind-whipped snow surface to sled down the slope on their bottoms. I followed, which made Lasti's eyes bug out as he worried I'd veer off course into a crater, or worse, to the right over the rocks.

A few more skids on my rear-feeling the cooling of my glutes that had worked hard and strong to get me there—and I arrived back at Stella Point. I thought it was time to rest again. I felt like a child with a near delirious mind. A high of accomplishment mixed with the oxygen-starved environment. My brain didn't seem hurried.

But in the game of getting down the mountain, each minute counts in getting an oxygen-starved climber to safety.

Now, Meke and Lasti seemed annoyed that we weren't taking the descent as seriously as we should. He never once hurried us on the way up. Now he wanted to get us down quickly.

I got up, with an "Ugh" of exhaustion. I felt spent—but it was 8:30 a.m. and our day of hiking had just begun.

The job ahead was to get back down to the Kibo Hut, have some snacks, rest for an hour or two and then climb down the other side of the mountain to the Horombo Huts. It would be just like the climb itinerary said—twelve to fifteen hours of hiking altogether. For once, I wished it was wrong, some kind of typo. We had spent the last eight hours in the most challenging environment that I had ever known. That meant at least four more hours of hiking. To have this ahead of me, even if it was downhill, was disheartening.

We would continue down the mountain at a much faster pace that we had gone up it. Speed walking was one of the things I wanted least to do at that point. Besides, my legs felt like Jell-O. I found myself clutching onto Lasti, who helped me keep a steady pace toward Gilman's Point on the way to the Jamaica Rocks, which seemed much more intimidating the second time around.

I wasn't the only one nearing a breaking point after the euphoric summit—Carla was too. After the rush down the slope on my rear, I saw her with Meke. She was a few steps past Stella Point, sitting.

"I'm so tired," she said. While the rest of the climbers, who were up and over Gilman's Point by then, were flush-faced, Carla was gaunt. Every part of her looked spent, and her rag doll arms flopped open with her poles still looped around to her wrists. She looked up at Meke, who helped her back to her feet.

Her boots were like giant ankle weights as she stepped f orward. The sun had been out for well over an hour now, making the perfectly manicured snow surface slick. One wrong step could lead down a crater slope or into a crash course with the exposed jagged volcanic rock.

Meke helped Carla. Lasti was my savior, safeguarding every step.

Chris was not far ahead. He stayed with us, sometimes moving down faster than me, but waiting for us to catch up.

This was no longer the familiar woods of New Jersey. This was rugged terrain, and this was why we had professionals with us. We gingerly made our way down the rocks. Now I wanted to rush, but with my trembling legs, I had to be careful not to stumble.

As the sun changed the terrain on top of the mountain, it also melted the ice holding the scree in place. The surface looked solid and sturdy but crushed under boot. This was an entirely different type of challenge on the mountain. This is why we needed to wear gaiters, a leg warmer-like sleeve between the ankle of our boots to our knees. If we didn't have them on properly, our footwear would fill with stone. There's a lot of trust involved in the art of scree running. You need to take a breath and let your body run down the mountain, falling as you may. So I lunged forward, with each step plunging into what was now like a vertical beach. Lasti and I were arm and arm down the mountain. My legs were limp as we tumbled at what felt like a breakneck pace down the mountain.

The scree that was once our sometimes solid surface was reduced to pebbles. We weren't on any path. We were heading down, like a chute of lava from this volcano. Sometimes we'd fall, tangled in each others' limbs. I apologized for my size, still feeling guilty Lasti was holding up such a large woman. He told me in Tanzania, big women were beautiful, and joked that he was the lucky one. I blushed. That was one of the few compliments I had ever had about beauty from someone other than Chris.

Meke, who held Carla on the way down, said, "Do you think her husband is jealous?"

"He's probably thankful," they laughed.

Right about then, Chris turned around and took a photo of us coming down the path.

It took an hour or two to make our way down the part of the mountain that took us six hours to hike up. Our tents were awaiting us. I could barely move and didn't want to as I struggled to pull myself in the tent, which had warmed in the sun. Chris and I peeled off our layers—down to our T-shirts—and hobbled in to rest for an hour before snack time. Stinky and soiled from head to toe—Chris and I kissed and held hands, laughing about the way down the mountain, so happy to have made it to the top. I fell asleep with a smile on my face.

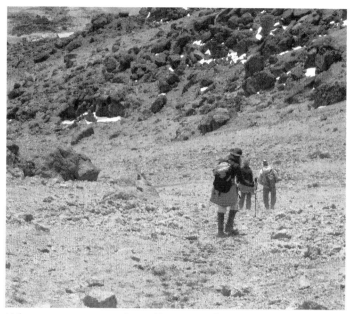

What goes up must go down. Trying to make our way down the unstable scree surface.

I was so grateful that I didn't have to use the toilet. That would have meant moving. But if I didn't have to use the bathroom, now six hours after my last bathroom break, I must be dehydrated. I looked at my CamelBak and realized it was mostly full. I pulled it up next to me, and started to chug it.

It can be hard to tell who will and who won't make it to Kilimanjaro's summit; the altitude and physical demands can prove too much, even for experienced climbers.

Meke confessed to me on the way down the mountain that most fat people don't summit. In fact, some porters were betting against me. On the way the down the mountain, most of our African Walking Company porters (who left camp an hour after we did and would arrive at our destination an hour before we

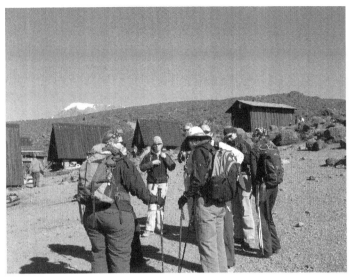

Gearing up for our last of hiking down the mountain.

did) passed and cheered, "Mama Kubwa!"

Porters from other climbing companies, lugging loads on their heads up the mountain, would ask Meke and Robbie how I did. They spoke in Swahili. Later, Robbie told me how each of the conversations went.

"Did she make it?"

"Yes, all the way to the top."

"Slowly, slowly?"

"No, she was strong the whole way," Robbie said.

18. THE LONG
WALK HOME

My hiking pants swished back and forth. It would take six hours and approximately thirteen miles to return to Marangu Gate, the trail's end. Even though our legs creaked as we rolled sleeping bags up one last time, the group hurried downward on the trail.

"Don't forget to look up," Ann reminded the group.

I obliged and right ahead, through a valley, was a silhouette of a mountain that looked almost identical to Camel's Hump. I turned back to tell Chris and then saw the ice cap of Kilimanjaro, stretching above its surrounding hills.

I thought about all the different things I would not have seen had I not decided to put one foot in front of the other. The Grand Canyon at sunrise and sunset, the silhouette of my hip bone that had been hidden for so many years, the loving smile of my husband as we journeyed the trails together and watched me fall in love with myself again.

There was sweat, a tumble or two, and maybe even a few torn pants along the way, but I had made it to the roof of Africa. There was no telling where I could go next.

Each step made me stronger. The destination was just part of the journey.

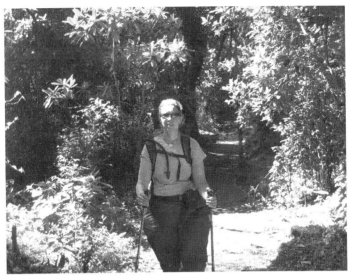

Enjoying the last little bit through the rain forest.

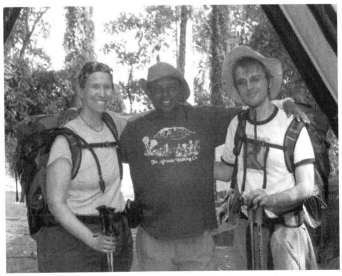

Me, Meke and Chris celebrating success at Kilimanjaro's gate.

EPILOGUE

When I came off the mountain, my friends asked what my next adventure would be. Rainier? Everest? Chris and I had another one in mind that would require a whole new set of gear and training. It was parenthood.

A few months after our return from Africa, I was pregnant. I caved to eating-for-two excuses. I had complications that made it difficult for me to walk across the living room. When our daughter was born almost exactly one year after our Kilimanjaro summit, I had sixty pounds to lose all over again.

As I struggled with being stuck between intention and action once again, I tried to remember what was so powerful about training for Kilimanjaro. I remembered how I was doing something I loved and was working for a cause bigger than myself.

I decided to make charity events that also kept me active my way of life. In 2009, I took on a fitness event for charity each month. I ended the year back on Kilimanjaro with a second fundraising hike for Global Alliance for Africa's AIDS orphans programs.

My journey has been up and down the scale since my first Kilimanjaro triumph. The most important thing I learned is to just keep moving forward.

ACTION
steps

1 GET YOUR BEARINGS
Talk to your doctor about your current physical state. Get an idea of what you can do and start doing it. You have to know where you are to know where you need to go.

2 LOOK BACK AND THEN MOVE FORWARD
We all have great and not-so-great life experiences. This is your life, not the life of others who have hurt you. Move forward with strength and purpose.

3 GO BEYOND THE NUMBER
Think about what you want to do, not what you want to weigh. Having a goal — from being able to walk around the block to doing a triathlon — gives you something real and tangible that you can visualize when it comes time to make everyday food or exercise choices.

4 FILL YOURSELF WITH PURPOSE
There are plenty of ways to keep your hands busy — and out of the cookie jar. Spend a few minutes writing Amnesty International letters on behalf of those whose human rights are violated or knit a blanket for a baby in need.

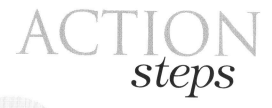

ACTION *steps*

5 GO OFF THE BEATEN PATH

Living on autopilot will get you nowhere. If you are looking to lose weight, think about what you should do differently. How can you shake things up — to eat lighter? How about your exercise routine—are you just going through the motions?

6 GET TO KNOW YOUR FOOD

Your food is your fuel — eat to power your body. Spend some time studying your food and what it does— and doesn't do — for you. From reading labels to asking how something is prepared at a restaurant — be an aware eater.

7 THINK BIG, START SMALL

Your journey begins now. Your weight gain was a result of many small decisions. Your weight loss will also be a result of many small decisions but you have to start somewhere.

8 GET A GUIDE

Any great adventure requires a great guide. Seek advice and help from those who are more experienced in your dream endeavor.

ACKNOWLEDGMENTS

Thank you to:

~ The more than 100 people who supported our Global Alliance for Africa fund-raising and training effort. Each one of you pushed me to the summit.

Global Alliance for Africa, especially Tom Derdak, for your amazing work with vulnerable children, and for allowing me to come on this journey with you.

~ Meke, Lasti, James, Robbie, Trophine and the wonderful African Walking Company staff who led us to the top of Mount Kilimanjaro. Without you, we would have been lost, really.

~ Ann, Sarah, Shawna, Lauren, Karen, Lisa and Carla for inspiring me with each step up the mountain.

~ My fitness instructors including Reina, Diane and Heather.

~ My Telluride altitude crew including Heather, Joanna, Dennis, Hawkeye and Rube.

~ My journalism mentors and colleagues for your patience and care over the years.

~ Leeza Hernandez for artfully designing this book.

~ My MediaBistro.com instructors and classmates for helping me find the words for this project.

~ Paula Derrow for being a champion for my story.

~ My parents and brothers for so much and my late grandmother Margaret for teaching me the power of my voice.

~ Robin and Jim for being amazing models for me in so many ways—from giving to grace.

Most of all, thank you to my husband, Chris, for being with me every step of the way, and to my daughter for inspiring me to keep moving forward.

RESOURCES & REFERENCES

Global Alliance for Africa ~ **www.globalallianceafrica.org**

Visit the website:
www.fatwomanonthemountain.com
to order journals, water bottles,
inspirational magnets and audio products.

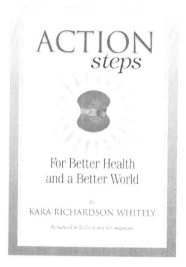

The website is a terrific resource for upcoming
webinars, seminars and other events.

Happy trails!

Kara

ABOUT THE AUTHOR

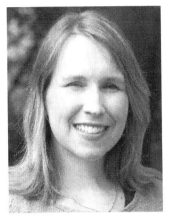

Kara Richardson Whitely takes action steps for health and a better world.

Her empowering story of going up mountains and down the scale has been featured in numerous blogs, radio programs, newspapers such as the *Tampa Tribune*, as well as *Self* and *Redbook* magazines. She is now planning a celebrity Kilimanjaro hike for charity in 2011 for a television series.

Kara has been a journalist for the past decade. She has written for numerous newspapers including the *Courier News*, *Ventura County Star*, the *Ann Arbor News*, the *Star-Ledger* as well as *Self*, *Every Day With Rachael Ray*, and *Runner's World* magazines.

Kara, who comes with the perspective of the two-thirds of Americans who are overweight or obese, is a national American Heart Association lifestyle change ambassador, sharing her story to inspire others to make positive lifestyle changes. She is a motivational speaker and has addressed audiences at events including the World Obesity Congress and Women's Health & Fitness Expo.

She is the founder of two websites:

www.fatwomanonthemountain.com and
www.savetheworldworkout.com.

She lives in Summit, New Jersey with her husband and two-year-old daughter, Anna.

Made in the USA
Charleston, SC
16 March 2011